T4-AVF-431

Judith Johnston

THINKING ABOUT CHILD LANGUAGE

Research to Practice

Thinking Publications University
A Division of Super Duper® Inc.
Greenville, South Carolina

© 2007 by Thinking Publications® University
© 2006 by Thinking Publications

Thinking Publications® University grants limited rights to individual professionals to reproduce and distribute pages that indicate duplication is permissible. Pages can be used for instruction only and must include Thinking Publications® University's copyright notice. All rights are reserved for pages without the permission-to-reprint notice. No part of these pages can be reproduced in any form, electronic or mechanical, including photocopy, recording, or any information storage and retrieval system, without permission in writing from the publisher.

11   10   09   08   07   06   8   7   6   5   4   3   2   1

Library of Congress Cataloging-in-Publication Data

Johnston, Judith R.
  Thinking about child language : research to practice / Judith Johnston
    p. ; cm.
  Contains updated and expanded essays previously published in The language intervention digest.
  Includes bibliographical references and indexes.
  ISBN 1-932054-45-6
  1. Language disorders in children. 2. Children--Language. 3. Language acquisition. I. Title
  [DNLM: 1. Language Disorders--diagnosis--Collected Works. 2. Language Therapy--Collected Works. 3. Child. 4. Language Development--Collected Works. WL 340.2 J72t 2006]
RJ496.L35J65 2006
618.92'855--dc22
                                                                    2005046631

Printed in the United States of America
Cover design by Nate Engen
Trademarks: All brand names and product names used in this book are the trade
              names, service marks, trademarks, or registered trademarks of their
              respective owners.

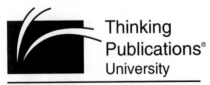

Thinking
Publications®
University

A Division of Super Duper® Inc.

Post Office Box 24997, Greenville, South Carolina 29616 USA
www.superduperinc.com • Call Toll Free 1-800-277-8737 • Fax Toll Free 1-800-978-7379
E-Mail: custserv@superduperinc.com

For my mothers.

They would have liked this book.

About the Author

Judith R. Johnston is a professor in the School of Audiology and Speech Sciences of the Faculty of Medicine at the University of British Columbia (UBC), and is known internationally for her expertise in developmental language disorders. Her extensive academic and clinical experience in both Canada and the United States has given her a broadly applicable perspective on intervention issues.

After receiving her bachelor of arts and master of arts degrees at Stanford University, Judith worked as a clinician at a rehabilitation center in San Mateo, California, and at the Institute for Childhood Aphasia at the Stanford Medical School. Hoping to clarify her understanding of the nature of intervention, she then completed doctoral studies in psychology at the University of California–Berkeley under the direction of Dan Slobin. While there, she served as a clinical and research consultant to the Richmond Unified Schools and the Los Angeles County Schools, and coordinated a large cross-linguistic study of language acquisition.

Judith began her academic career in 1977 at Indiana University Bloomington, and remained there until 1988. She then joined the faculty at UBC as Director of the School of Audiology and Speech Sciences.

Judith's research has focused on the developmental relationships between language and cognition, particularly as seen in the profiles of children with specific language impairments. She was one of the first researchers to show that such children also have difficulties with nonverbal tasks, and to argue that the total evidence picture indicates limitations in cognitive processing capacity. Her work has been published in over one hundred professional and scientific articles, proceedings, and book chapters.

Judith is also known as a committed teacher and mentor whose former students are professional and scientific leaders across North America. Her scholarship and teaching have been recognized in numerous awards, most recently the Honors of the American Speech-Language-Hearing Association, and the 3M Teaching Fellowship given by the Canadian Society for Teaching and Learning in Higher Education.

Contents

Contents

Contents

Preface

I have been a speech-language pathologist and teacher of speech-language pathologists for almost 40 years, specializing in early language intervention. Ours is a demanding profession. Relevant information pours at us from all directions—neurology, genetics, acoustics, psychology, linguistics, education. We must stay open to new ideas and be eager to acquire new skills, while at the same time remaining grounded in explicit and well-considered views about the general nature of the human 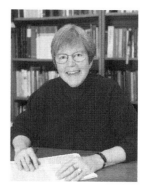 mind and language. Perhaps the greatest challenge of all is that our profession never allows us to wait until we are sure. Instead, we must learn to read wisely, weigh the evidence, consider the consequences, choose the best-bet course of action, and stay attentive to outcomes. Each decision leads to new questions, and the exploring and thinking begins anew. For me, this is the real continuing education—the self-guided learning that is inherent in good practice. Rather than see it as a burden, I choose to see it as an adventure and opportunity. How fortunate we are to be in a field that welcomes creative thinking and new knowledge at every turn.

This collection of essays is a distillation of what I have learned, and continue to learn, as I read new research studies and think about their application to practice. The essays are not comprehensive reviews of evidence but are my organized reflections on topics of clinical relevance. Each essay originally appeared online, as an issue of *The Language Intervention Digest*. The set included in this book was written between March of 2002 and December of 2004, and each one begins with summaries of a research article or two that first appeared during, or close to, this period. The summaries are followed by a general commentary and a discussion of clinical applications that reflect the decades that I have spent thinking and talking about early language intervention. The material in the essays was written initially for speech-language pathologists, but language specialists from other disciplines (e.g., special education, early childhood education, clinical linguistics, or second language learning) should also find much that is relevant to their educational practice.

The essays are written informally, and can be read in the breathing spaces of a busy day. The ideas within the essays are, however, far from casual. They are meant to be chewed on, talked about, responded to. They deal, not with some ivory tower reality, but with the everyday challenges of language intervention. I hope you will find them easy to understand and hard to ignore. I also hope that, by the time the last essay has been read, you will have acquired the models and inspiration you need to continue turning research into practice.

For this book presentation, the essays have been reorganized, updated, and expanded with a new set of learning tools. At the end of most of the essays you will find a list of additional readings, a set of questions for use in workplace or classroom discussion groups, and one or more small experiments or investigations that you could carry out to further explore the ideas contained therein. Taken together, the essays and activities are not meant to provide solutions to clinical problems, but to identify issues and help you create your own answers. You may find you disagree with some or many of my conclusions. That is fine; good practice requires only that you be informed and thoughtful.

I'm the first to admit that this is an unusual book, one that may take some getting used to. I set out to create a feast of ideas, but true to my Swedish heritage, I seem to have created a smorgasbord. There is a great variety of dishes, carefully arranged, with all the herring at one end of the table and the cheeses at the other. The pleasures of a smorgasbord, however, depend not only on what is on the plates, but also on knowing how to make a good meal. You should take small portions of whatever appeals, keep coming back for more, and expect to find things that you missed the first time around.

That is exactly the way to approach this book. Here you will find a wide array of short, clinically relevant essays, arranged by general topic area. They can be read in any order, according to your curiosities and needs. You may even decide that some of the essays invite a second reading as your own experience highlights new aspects of a topic.

In the back of the book you will find a number of items to help you make your way. There is a chart indicating the pertinent developmental levels and language domains for each essay (Appendix A) and a list of the various websites mentioned throughout the book (Appendix B). When standardized tests are mentioned in the essays, I use their abbreviated titles; you will find the full title, citation, and a description for each in Appendix C. Appendix D provides a description of the language analysis software program, Systematic Analysis of Language Transcripts (SALT; Miller & Iglesias, 2003–2005), which is mentioned in many of the essays. Finally, Appendix E consists of question sets and exercises written for students who are preparing to be speech-language pathologists and do not yet have much clinical experience. Following the appendices, you will find a glossary, an author index, and a subject index. Remember to check these resources when you meet an unfamiliar term, or are looking for ideas on a particular topic. I have shortened the citation of names in the essays, but all authors for each citation are found in the author index and the reference list.

Throughout the book, the Questions for Discussion and Thought are marked with a talking stick. In wide use by native peoples throughout North America, talking sticks made of various materials were used to assist group process. During any important discussion, the "stick" would be systematically passed from person to person, to ensure that everyone who wished to make a contribution could do so. It also served as a visible reminder to listeners that it was their duty to pay close attention to the ideas being expressed. Since one root of my family tree lies in the Cherokee Nation, this symbol seemed like a good way to remind readers that good discussion requires a commitment to inclusion and shared responsibility.

At the time this book went to press, a number of options for using the essays to earn continuing education units were under consideration. Interested readers should visit the Thinking Publications website (www.ThinkingPublications.com) for information on where and how to access a CEU option.

It is impossible to mention all the people and events that have shaped my thinking about intervention over the past 40 years. I have been extraordinarily fortunate to have spent my professional life in the company of fine scholars, clinicians, and friends. There are a group of colleagues I would like to thank for their specific help in preparing this book, as critics, readers, listeners, and assistants: Kate Ballem, Penny Boyes-Braem, Monique Charest, Paola Colozzo, Ron Gillam, Jeanette Leonard, Jon Miller, Rachael Moser, Sheri Milham, and Jo Nussbaum. Their efforts and enthusiasm kept me moving along. Thanks go to the field reviewers for their helpful comments: Barbara L. Brown, Janet Harrison, Laura Hurd, and Vicki Lord Larson. I would also like to thank Carolyn Johnson and colleagues at the UBC School of Audiology and Speech Sciences for supporting my initial vision for *The Language Intervention Digest,* and the readers of the *Digest* for their commitment to learning. And finally, a heartfelt thank you to my project editor, Joyce Olson, for patience, flexibility, and expertise; to Nate Engen and Dathan Boardman for art; to Jan Carroll for technical editing; and to all the folks at Thinking Publications for respecting, and fostering, intelligent practice.

Foundations of Practice

My father was a structural engineer, so on occasion our dinner conversation turned to soil quality, pile drivers, and the importance of a good foundation. As speech-language pathologists (SLPs) and language specialists, we are constantly building the edifice of practice. The strength and integrity of our work will, like a house, depend on its foundation. To be sure, effective intervention demands much knowledge about language disorders, about assessment procedures and flow charts, and about therapeutic frameworks and activities. But behind this visibly professional expertise there is also the need for the basic theories and thinking tools that can serve as our foundation.

The essays in this section consider four of the pillars that support our intervention decisions. First, there is our knowledge of the principles and facts of normal language learning. Before we can facilitate a child's language growth, we need to understand how children learn to talk and what they must learn in order to be effective communicators. Secondly, there is the pillar of critical appraisal. We constantly hear about new clinical programs and read research studies about intervention outcomes. This information must be systematically evaluated and integrated with prior knowledge. In order to do so we need to understand research design and be able to weigh the evidence. Given our complex scope of practice, we don't yet have strong or clear answers to many of our clinical questions. Much remains empirically uncertain. Our third pillar, then, is a set of strategies that can help us make decisions in spite of uncertainty—strategies such as cost/benefit analysis in which we compare the consequences of our various possible actions. The fourth and final pillar is an appreciation of the limits of science. All human activity reflects values and beliefs as well as facts. Sculptors, lawyers, grocery clerks, chemists, and SLPs—we all select, prioritize, and interpret the events of our lives. This reality invites us to be conscious of our own values and respectful of others, and finally to acknowledge our common humanity with wisdom and compassion. Most of this book is about the particulars of early language intervention, but it seemed important to include at least a few thoughts about foundations.

1 Factors That Influence Language Development

Learning to talk is one of the most visible and important achievements of early childhood. In a matter of months, and without explicit teaching, toddlers move from hesitant single words to fluent sentences, and from a small vocabulary to one that is growing by six new words a day. New language tools mean new opportunities for social understanding; for learning about the world; and for sharing experiences, pleasures, and needs.

The Nature of Language Knowledge

Language development is even more impressive when we consider the nature of what is learned. It may seem that children merely need to remember what they hear and repeat it at some later time. But as Chomsky (1959) pointed out so many years ago, if this were the essence of language learning, we would not be successful communicators. Verbal communication requires productivity, that is, the ability to create an infinite number of utterances we have never heard before. This endless novelty requires that some aspects of language knowledge be abstract. Ultimately, "rules" for combining words cannot be rules about particular words, but must be rules about classes of words such as nouns, verbs, or prepositions. Once these abstract blueprints are available, the speaker can fill the "slots" in a sentence with the words that best convey the message of the moment. Chomsky's key point was that since abstractions cannot ever be directly experienced, they must emerge from the child's own mental activity as he or she listens to speech.

The Debate

The nature of the mental activity that underlies language learning is widely debated among child language experts. One group of theorists argues that language input merely triggers grammatical knowledge that is already genetically available (Pinker, 1984). The opposition argues that grammatical knowledge results from the way the human mind analyzes and organizes information and is not innate (Elman et al., 1996). This debate reflects fundamentally different beliefs about human development and is not likely to be resolved. However, there are at least two areas in which there is a substantial consensus that can guide educators and

3

policymakers: (1) the predictability of the course of language acquisition and (2) its multideterminate nature.

The Common Ground

Predictable Sequences and Determining Factors

In broad stroke, the observable facts of language development are not in dispute. Most children begin speaking during their second year and by age 2 are likely to know at least 50 words and to be combining them into short phrases (Rescorla, 1989). When vocabulary size reaches about 200 words, the rate of word learning increases dramatically and grammatical-function words such as articles and prepositions begin to be used with some consistency (Bates & Goodman, 1997). During the preschool years, sentence patterns become increasingly complex and vocabulary diversifies to include relational terms that express notions of size, location, quantity, and time (Clark, 1993). By the age of 4;6 or so, most children have acquired the basic grammar of the sentence (Paul, 1981). From that point onward, children learn to use language more efficiently and more effectively. They also learn how to create and maintain larger language units such as conversation or narrative (Owens, 2001). Although there are individual differences in rate of development, the sequence in which various forms appear is highly predictable both within and across stages (Crystal et al., 1976).

There is also considerable agreement that the course of language development reflects the interplay of factors in at least five domains: social, perceptual, cognitive processes, conceptual, and linguistic. Theorists differ in the emphasis and degree of determination posited for a given domain, but most would agree that each is relevant. There is a large body of research supporting the view that language learning is influenced by many aspects of human experience and capability. I'll mention two findings in each area that capture the flavor of the available evidence.

Social

1. **Toddlers infer a speaker's communicative intent.** They can use that information to guide their language learning. For example, as early as 24 months, they are able to infer solely from an adult's excited tone of voice and from the physical setting, that a new word must refer to an object that has been placed on the table while the adult was away (Akhtar et al., 1996).

2. **The verbal environment influences language learning.** Between the ages of 1 and 3, children from highly verbal "professional" families hear nearly three times as many words per week as children from low verbal "welfare" families. Longitudinal data show that aspects of this early *parental* language predict language scores at age 9 (Hart & Risley, 1995).

Perceptual

1. **Infant perception sets the stage.** Auditory perceptual skills at 6 or 12 months of age can predict vocabulary size and syntactic complexity at 23 months of age (Trehub & Henderson, 1996).

2. **Perceptibility matters.** In English, the forms that are challenging for impaired learners are forms with reduced perceptual salience, such as those that are unstressed (e.g., the auxiliary verb *is)* or those that may lie within a consonant cluster (e.g., the past tense *-ed* in *walked;* Leonard, 1992).

Cognitive Processes

1. **Frequency affects rate of learning.** Children who hear an unusually high proportion of examples of a language form learn that form faster than children who receive ordinary input (Nelson et al., 1996).

2. **Tradeoffs can occur among the different domains of language.** This happens when the total targeted sentence requires more mental resource than the child has available. For example, children make more errors on small grammatical forms such as verb endings and prepositions in sentences with complex syntax than in sentences with simple syntax (Namazi & Johnston, 1997).

Conceptual

1. **Relational terms are linked to mental age.** Words that express notions of time, causality, location, size, and order are correlated with mental age much more than words that simply refer to objects and events (Fazio et al., 1993). Moreover, children learning different languages learn to talk about spatial locations such as *in* or *next to* in much the same order, regardless of the grammatical devices of their particular language (Johnston & Slobin, 1979).

2. **Language skills are affected by world knowledge.** Children understand sentences with *because* or *so* better if the content concerns familiar events

such as birthday parties than if the content concerns unfamiliar events such as changing the tire on a car (Johnston & Welsh, 2000).

Linguistic

1. **Verb endings are cues to verb meaning.** If a new verb ends in -*ing*, three-year-olds learning English will decide that it refers to an *activity* such as *swim,* rather than to a *completed change of state* such as *push off* (Carr & Johnston, 2001). Essay 32 elaborates on this point.

2. **Current vocabulary influences new learning.** Toddlers usually decide that a new word refers to the object for which they do not already have a label (Clark, 1993).

Nature and Nurture

These are just some of the findings that, taken together, speak convincingly of the interactive nature of development. Children come to the task of language learning with perceptual mechanisms that function in a certain way and with finite attention and memory capacities. These cognitive systems will, at the least, influence what is noticed in the language input, and may well be central to the learning process. Similarly, children's prior experience with the material and social world provides the early bases for interpreting the language around them. Later, they also will make use of language cues. The course of language acquisition is not, however, driven exclusively from within. The structure of the language to be learned, and the frequency with which various forms are heard, will also have an effect. Despite the theoretical debates, it seems clear that language skills reflect knowledge and capabilities in virtually every domain and should not be viewed in an insular fashion.

Educational and Policy Implications

Educators and policymakers have often ignored the preschooler whose language seems to be lagging behind development in other areas, arguing that such children are "just a bit late" in talking. The research evidence suggests instead that language acquisition should be treated as an important barometer of success in complex integrative tasks. Whenever language "fails," other domains are implicated as well—as either causes or consequences. Indeed, major epidemiological studies have now demonstrated that children diagnosed with specific language disorders at age 4 are at high risk for academic failure and mental health problems well into young adulthood (Beitchman et al., 2001; Young et al., 2002). Fortunately, the research evidence also indicates that it is possible to accelerate language learning (Nye et al., 1987). Even though the child must be the one to create the abstract patterns from the language data, we can facilitate this learning (1) by presenting language examples that are in accord with the child's perceptual, social, and cognitive resources, and (2) by choosing learning goals that are in harmony with the common course of development.❖

Johnston, J. (2005). Factors that influence language development. In R. Tremblay, R. Barr & R. Peters (Eds.), *Encyclopedia on Early Childhood Development [online]*. Montreal, Quebec: Centre for Excellence for Early Child Development; 2005:1–6/ Available at http://www.excellence-earlychildhood.ca/documents/Johnston ANGxp.pdf. Accessed July, 2005.

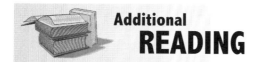

Additional READING

Tomasello, M. (Ed.). (2003). *The new psychology of language: Cognitive and functional approaches to language structure, Vol 2*. Mahwah, NJ: Earlbaum.

NOTE: This volume contains a number of chapters that enrich our understanding of the social and cognitive contexts of language learning. Note in particular chapters by Talmay, Kemmer, and Bybee.

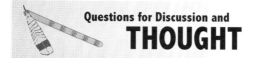

Questions for Discussion and THOUGHT

1. This essay was written for educators and policymakers. How would you alter it for a group of parents at a daycare center? Would you make different points? Use different illustrations?

2. Do you think there is a connection between the factors described on pages 4 to 6 and the predictable language sequences described on pages 3 and 4?

3. Broadly sketched, there are two main theoretical perspectives on language acquisition these days: (1) the Innate Account that posits a genetically provided grammar and an acquisition process that triggers this knowledge, and (2) the Connectionist (or Cognitivist) Account that posits a genetically provided set of learning mechanisms that record, organize, and abstract from world experience. Which position best reflects your own perspective on language learning? Could an observer infer your theoretical views by watching your therapy session?

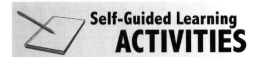 **Self-Guided Learning ACTIVITIES**

1. Review the list of factors with their supporting evidence. Which ones are you most and least familiar with? Take the one that you feel least knowledgeable about, find a language acquisition textbook (On your bookshelf? In your public library?), and read the pertinent sections.

2. Review the list of factors and evidence and then think about its implications for parent-child interaction. Create a five-point sheet of advice to parents.

2 Evidence? What Evidence?

There is much talk about evidence-based practice in the SLP literature these days. Initially, this phrase brought to mind stories about the emperor's new clothes and tempests in teapots. Of course we should base our practice on the evidence, and we do. So what's all the fuss? I have to admit, however, that the more I think about this topic, the more interesting it becomes. The real question is not whether we should base our practice on the evidence, but rather what sort of evidence should we use? And where can we find it?

What Sort of Evidence?

I'll begin with the first question: What sort of evidence should we use? Good evidence is evidence that (1) comes from studies with strong designs, (2) can be readily interpreted, and (3) is up-to-date. An Oxford study of physicians' treatment decisions indicated that some 82 percent were supported by this sort of high quality evidence (Ellis et al., 1995). How well do we do?

Strong Evidence

Evidence about a clinical practice can be graded according to its strength, that is, according to the degree to which it can reliably indicate that a practice has an effect, and that this effect can be replicated and generalized. Table 2.1 on page 10 ranks various research designs according to the strength of the evidence they yield, in descending order of strength.

The ranking in this table is a reworded and condensed version of the scheme used by the Centre for Evidence-Based Medicine at Oxford University. The full scheme is one of the most comprehensive of those in current use, and includes quality judgments and rankings for clinical activities other than therapy such as screening or diagnosis. The ultimate goal is to evaluate bodies of research considered as a whole, and determine the highest level, range of levels, or average level of evidence in support of a given practice.

Let's begin with the first part of the evaluation, and use the ranks in Table 2.1 to evaluate the evidence that supports some of the typical practices in early language intervention. First, consider the use of total communication (sign or gesture plus speech) to assist hearing children with the initial stages of language learning. Goodwyn and Acredolo (1993) provide supporting evidence at Level 3 for

Research Designs for Studies of Therapy
Ranked by Strength of Evidence

Table 2.1

Rank	Design
1	Meta-analysis of controlled and randomized experimental studies
2	Well-designed, controlled, and randomized experimental study
3	Well-designed group comparison study with controls but no randomization
4	Well-designed quasi-experimental (observational) study
5	Well-designed single-subject study with controls
6	Case studies and correlational designs
7	Opinions of respected authorities based on clinical experience, or reports of expert committees

Source: Ball et al. (2001)

normally developing children, and there is additional positive evidence from Ellis Weismer and Hesketh (1993) with disordered children, also at Level 3. In regard to the use of another common clinical practice, focused expansions, we have Fey et al. (1993), Nelson et al. (1996), and a scatter of earlier studies that provide evidence at Levels 2 and 3.

What about the use of telegraphic speech as the input for language learners at early stages of language? This is a widely used practice and I suspect many of us can remember playing with a young child and saying things like, "Up. More up" or "Daddy go" or "Dolly out." A colleague here at UBC recently spent five months looking for evidence on this practice, and discovered that as far as she could ascertain, it had never been evaluated with a clinical sample. What little evidence she could find was only at Level 7. Take a moment to think about other intervention techniques that you use in your language therapy sessions. Do you use written word cues? Do you take your therapy into the classroom? Do you use parent groups? Ratings of the evidence for these three practices are listed on page 16 following the learning activities at the end of the essay.

Interpretable Evidence

In addition to evaluating the strength of the evidence, we need to think carefully about what each piece of evidence really concerns. This sounds more straightforward than it is. A report by Howard Goldstein (2002) regarding treatment efficacy in communication intervention for children with autism will illustrate the challenges. Goldstein reviewed 20 years of peer-reviewed research, and found 60 studies that provided evidence, albeit at Levels 5 and 6. While the evidence in any one of these studies is relatively weak, there is good agreement in the findings, which strengthens the general conclusion that children with autism improve their communication patterns following intervention. The problem here is that the interventions being evaluated were both diverse and underspecified. Milieu Therapy, Discrete Trial Learning, and the use of sign language all led to significant treatment effects. However, since the therapies were presented as packages, we don't know which features of the various programs were critical, nor do we know their relative effectiveness. In short, we have evidence, but it does not yet point to best practice.

As a second example, recall what you know of the literature on elicited imitation. Several studies with strong Level 2 or 3 designs have compared the outcomes of this procedure with the outcomes from focused modeling, and report that elicited imitation is more effective (e.g., Cole & Dale, 1986; Connell & Stone, 1992). There is also a very large body of older literature showing that elicited imitation procedures led to treatment effects in persons with severe mental retardation. Evidence in these studies tends to be at only Level 5 or 6, but again the outcomes are generally positive. Note, however, that all of these studies have compared elicited imitation techniques with techniques that require no talking at all. So, is this evidence about elicited imitation or about the importance of some sort of practice in actually producing the new form? An almost forgotten study by Ellis Weismer and Murray-Branch (1989) suggests the latter. These researchers compared focused modeling with evoked production, the creation of contexts that invite repetitive use of a targeted language form without making children repeat the therapist's utterances. The sample size was small, and the level of evidence was only at Level 5, but the outcomes indicated that *evoked production* was the more effective approach. It well may be that research findings that are usually cited to support the use of elicited imitation should be reinterpreted merely as evidence that children learn better when they need to actually produce the new form. The critical study comparing elicited imitation with evoked production has yet to be done.

Up-to-Date Evidence

Although the flow of language intervention research is regrettably slow, new studies *do* continue to appear, and some of them require us to revise our practice guidelines. The evidence attesting to the efficacy of parent education programs was for some years weak at best. The few experimental studies (Level 3 or 4) that had been done had failed to indicate any effect of therapy, and only the opinions of experts (Level 7) indicated that this approach was viable. Then, three studies by Fey et al. (1993), Girolametto et al. (1996), and Parsons (1991) provided strong Level 2 and 3 evidence that if parent education programs were individualized, they could be effective. These studies led me to a new view of evidence-based practice in the area of parent programming. Note that when there is only a small amount of evidence available on a given practice, even 2 or 3 new studies can change the bottom line conclusion.

Where Do We Find the Evidence?

I'm sure there is more to be said about the nature of the evidence that should underlie our practice, but at least we can be looking for good design, clarity, and currency. Where do we find such evidence? The most compelling information will come from review articles, with or without quantitative meta-analysis. If review articles are not available, we will need to consult the primary research literature ourselves. A half day in a college or university library would provide ample time to do computer-based searches for the year's intervention research. I would suggest using the *PsychInfo* indexes. This service covers books, book chapters, and almost all of the journals that would report research of interest. You can limit your search by the age of the children, and specifically ask for reports of treatment effects or for reviews. If there does not seem to be any intervention research that addresses the therapy approach or procedure you are interested in, you could also seek information about normal patterns of development, and use those as an initial guide to practice. For example, there are useful articles in the child language literature on the role of imitation in language learning that can help us make decisions about the use of elicited imitation procedures. (Those of you who do not have access to a university library could try an Internet search with Google Scholar, or could subscribe to a professional bibliographic service.)

There are several national and international groups that collaborate in the publishing of evidence-based practice reviews. The most well-known of these is the

Cochrane Collaboration, an independent, nonprofit group that specializes in best practice reviews for the healthcare sector. One thing to keep in mind as you read reviews by this and other groups is that they often set the minimum level of acceptable evidence very high, at Level 1 or 2. Such evidence is indeed strong and in some cases preferable, but it may not be the most appropriate standard in speech-language pathology. Until recently, our intervention research typically measured and compared language progress in treatment and no-treatment groups. For various ethical and logistical reasons, random assignment to these groups was not possible, limiting our highest evidence to Level 3. If you read a medically oriented review and the reviewer concludes that there is no evidence that speech-language therapy works with a particular population, this may only mean that there is no evidence at Level 1 or 2. There may be quite convincing evidence at Level 3, which I would accept as adequate for many of the treatment decisions we make.

This problem will decrease as language intervention research shifts to comparisons of two or more therapy procedures. For this type of question, random assignment to treatment groups is ethical and possible since we often cannot know a priori which treatment is best. This fact may allow us to create more evidence at the highest levels. However, randomized groups must be quite large to allow control of the many child factors determining outcomes, and this fact may continue to limit the feasibility of Level 1 and 2 designs. Researchers do not move immediately to large-sample, randomized clinical trials since this sort of project makes large demands on time and money. Preliminary, smaller-sample studies must usually pave the way. This means that the maturity of a line of investigation also needs to be taken into account when deciding on the value of evidence. Results from a case study or a small-sample investigation have more value if they concern a new line of inquiry than if a larger body of studies already exists.

Where does the Internet figure in the evidence picture? There are very few on-line treatment guidelines for specific sorts of children with communication disorders. Much of what the search engine finds is at a level of evidence that doesn't even appear on the Oxford list, namely the opinions of individual clinicians without expert credentials. The important exception to this rule are the websites of organizations that sponsor and archive systematic review papers. At least two of these groups focus on educational issues: the What Works Clearinghouse (http://w-w-c.org) and The Campbell Collaboration (www.campbellcollaboration.org).

Internet resources should rapidly improve since many professional organizations and agencies are planning to post treatment guidelines. The American Speech-Language-Hearing Association has begun an effort to generate best practice review papers, and their website should prove useful (www.asha.org). A second valuable initiative was begun in the spring of 2004 when the Bamford-Lahey Foundation supported a meeting of child language intervention researchers to discuss evidence-based practice. The website of the foundation has a record of these deliberations as well as a set of resource materials. It will also post any review papers on practices in developmental language intervention that are written by members of this group (www.bamford-lahey.org). As you follow these and similar initiatives, just remember to consider the source.

How Well Do We Do?

I suspect that most speech-language pathologists do not yet have strong evidence for 82 percent of their treatment decisions. This may just mean that the practice is untested, rather than that it is useless or unwise. However, I'm afraid that it also reflects the fact that we seldom evaluate our practices in a systematic fashion. If we are to provide the highest quality care, our clinical decisions must reflect an integration of "current high quality research evidence...with practitioner expertise and client preferences and values" (ASHA, 2005b, p.1).

I now see evidence-based practice as a great goal for our maturing profession. Both individually and collectively, we need to make a list of the procedures and decision rules we commonly use in language intervention. Then, for each item on the list, we need to ascertain the source and strength of the available evidence. This would be a fair-sized undertaking and one which would need some time, but the product of this exercise would be invaluable. It would indicate which aspects of our practice have a record of proven efficacy, and which ones require further refinement or have yet to be studied. We may even find a few practices that can be set aside as a waste of time. At the very least, the process of considering the evidence would sharpen our thinking about practice patterns and help us discover opportunities for improvement.❖

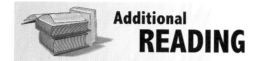

**Additional
READING**

Dollaghan, C. (2004, April 13). Evidence-based practice: Myths and realities. The ASHA Leader, 12, 4–5.

There is also a growing number of online resources for clinicians who want to learn more about evaluating clinical evidence. Two such sites are the Centre for Evidence-Based Medicine at the University of Toronto (www.cebm.utoronto.ca), especially the section entitled "Practicing EBM," and the Centre for Evidence-Based Medicine at Oxford University noted earlier (www.cebm.net).

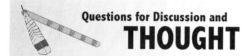

**Questions for Discussion and
THOUGHT**

1. Not all of the experts in language intervention research would agree with the order of the items on the Oxford ladder of evidence. The debate focuses on the relative value of studies with single-subject designs, Levels 5 and 6. What are the strengths and weaknesses of these designs? Would you place these studies somewhere else on the ladder?

2. What are the practices that you most wish someone would study? Try to list them with a high degree of specificity. For example: What is the effect of teaching a nonverbal autistic child to use picture symbols to request objects or actions? Does the rate of communicative acts increase? Does the family report fewer episodes of upset? Is the child more likely to acquire speech?

3. Even when there is strong evidence in support of a particular intervention practice, the SLP or language specialist must decide whether it is relevant to a particular client. What characteristics or factors should be considered?

Self-Guided Learning
ACTIVITIES

1. Consider one 30-minute session of direct language intervention with an individual child that you conducted within the past week. Make a list of two or three of the techniques, procedures, or strategies that you used during the session. Then, try to remember when and where you learned each of them, and whether you have read or heard about any research studies or expert opinion that support its use.

2. Here are reports of two research studies on similar topics, one with a single-subject design and one with a group design. Read the two articles and then reconsider your answers to the first Question for Discussion and Thought (page 15).

> Ellis Weismer, S. E., & Murray-Branch, J. (1989). Modeling versus modeling-plus evoked production training: A comparison of two language intervention methods. Journal of Speech and Hearing Disorders, 54, 269–281.

> Nelson, K. E., Camarata, S. M., Welsh, J., Butkovsky, L., & Camarata, M. (1996). Effects of imitative and conversational recasting treatment on the acquisition of grammar in children with specific language impairment and younger language-normal children. Journal of Speech and Hearing Research, 39, 850–859.

Here are the answers to the questions regarding Level of Evidence as of October, 2004: Written word cues—Level 7; Therapy in the classroom—one study at Level 4; Parent groups—Level 2, but only for earliest stages of language.

3 Doing What Works

Each year I teach an introductory course on developmental language intervention, and the first topic is always "Dealing with Uncertainty." As they read the literature on intervention studies, my students understand why I begin that way. Even if we consider only those studies that report significant intervention effects, the variety in method and approach is astounding: dramatic play, toy demonstrations, parent education, picture labeling, conversational expansions, imitative drills, metalinguistic analyses. The settings and change agents vary as well: parents at home, peers at preschool, SLPs in school broom closets. My students quite reasonably want to know how to decide among these various methods. And so do I.

It is a bit disconcerting, isn't it? The practical genes that got us into the SLP business in the first place would find such satisfaction in just "doing what works." But it turns out that this practical rule doesn't get us very far. Many things "work." While that is in its own way reassuring, it doesn't help us make therapy plans. The problem with the intervention research is that most studies have only compared the progress of children in a given intervention to the progress of children receiving no treatment at all. What we need now are more of the comparative studies that move beyond mere efficacy to determine which sort of therapy works best? For whom? Why? And over what time period?

Goal Attack Strategies

Ann Tyler and her colleagues (2003) report one such comparative study. Let me set the stage for their work by telling you about Chris. Picture a totally engaging five-year-old in bib overalls talking about his family's hunting trip. He describes the long car ride, the rifle, and the white mountain sheep with long curled horns. He explains that the family went, not to the regular mountains, but to ones that look "like this," and recreates a high peak silhouette with careful gestures. When the SLP asks him what they did with the sheep, Chris explains "/iɛɪə'ʌ/." The SLP scrambles valiantly but it is three or four turns before she determines that the /ʌ/ is in fact a sheepskin rug.

Chris had obvious phonological difficulties, severe enough that it was five more years before he acquired the /r/. But he also fell far below age expectations in grammatical complexity, and this fact raised the question of what area to tackle first: phonology or morphosyntax? There is a good case to be made in each direction. The meaning distinctions encoded with bound morphemes such as the -*ed* or -*s* could provide the motive for phonological growth. Or, the ability to produce word-final consonant clusters could enable morphological marking.

Research studies have demonstrated both patterns of influence. Tyler and Sandoval (1994), for example, report morphological gains following phonological training with a controlled, small sample. Tyler et al. (2002) report that morphological intervention led to phonological gains in a large group of preschoolers. So which domain should be targeted first and for how long? Fey (1986) refers to this aspect of intervention planning as *goal attack strategies* and describes various options. For example, the SLP can focus on one learning goal until some performance level criterion is reached and then move to another, or the SLP can focus on several learning goals in the same session, either simultaneously or in sequence, and either related to each other or not.

Ann Tyler and colleagues (2003) decided to test the relative efficacy of four goal attack strategies for children who, like Chris, have both morphosyntactic and phonological difficulties. Forty children, ages 3 to 6, were randomly assigned to one of four therapy programs differing only in the sequence and timing of the targeted learning goals:

- 12 weeks of work on morphosyntax followed by 12 weeks on phonology

- 12 weeks of work on phonology followed by 12 weeks on morphosyntax

- 24 weeks alternating between work on morphosyntax and on phonology

- 24 weeks of simultaneous work on the two areas, *within* activities

There was also a control group drawn from children on school and clinic waiting lists.

Therapy sessions were held twice a week for a total of 75 minutes, half with children individually and half with children in groups of three. The sessions were designed such that comparable numbers of models (75–80 per session) and opportunities for production (23 per session) were provided in each condition. The therapy approach for both the phonological and the morphosyntactic goals was hybrid (Fey, 1986), in that it made use of structured activities but fairly natural language. In order to compare the effects of the four strategies, children were assessed prior to the program, and again at 12 and at 24 weeks. At each test point, data were collected from language samples and from a standard test of speech sound production. The actual indices used to determine efficacy were highly focused: percentage correct use for finite verb morphology (combining past tense, third person singular, and all BE forms), and percentage correct for test items requiring use of the child's speech sound targets.

Here's what Tyler and her colleagues found:

- Children receiving therapy did make more progress than the control group for both morphosyntactic and phonological goals.

- Gains in some conditions were much greater than in others. It was children in the alternating-weeks condition who showed the most improvement in finite verb morphology, by a factor of 2:1 by the end of the program. Gains in phonology, on the other hand, were equivalent for the four groups. This was true even at 12 weeks when we might have expected greater gains for children who had only received phonological therapy.

The alternating-weeks strategy has good intuitive appeal. It seems reasonable that this would be the best way to maximize cross-domain influences in both directions. However, if reciprocal facilitation were really occurring, the phonological gains should have been higher in the alternating-weeks condition as well, and they weren't. There was also no evidence that phonological training affected morphosyntax in any way. These two facts suggest that the alternating nature of the third condition was not the feature that made it so effective. Instead, it was probably the facts that morphosyntax was spread throughout the entire 24-week period and was addressed in focused activities that made the difference.

Whatever the reason, I was ready to recommend use of the alternating goal attack strategy for children like Chris when I noticed one further fact about this study. Individual goals had been established for each child based on their first assessment. It turns out that none of the children needed work on word final /s/, /z/, /d/, or /t/. Moreover, only six children showed final consonant cluster deletion/reduction. Since there is little reason to expect that work on /l/, /f/, or /k/ would lead to improvements in finite verb morphology, the failure to find this effect is not surprising. More importantly, we don't know now whether the alternating strategy would be best for children like Chris whose phonological difficulties do include final consonant deletion and speech sounds that occur in verb endings. It remains possible that phonological work would promote morphosyntax for these children and hence should be scheduled first.

This study is a strong exemplar of the comparative studies now being done. The design and implementation are excellent, yielding a strong level of evidence. For children with phonological problems not directly related to verb morphology, it does seem that the alternating goal attack strategy is a good idea. Work on morphosyntax could be alternated with work on pragmatics, vocabulary, or sentence patterns as well as with work on phonology. For children like Chris, however, the question remains unanswered. Tyler and her colleagues plan to explore goal attack strategies further in future studies. Unlike the researchers, we must make our decisions now, in the absence of clear findings, because the children won't wait.

When Even the New Facts Fail: Three Strategies for Dealing with Uncertainty

Language therapy deals with the human mind and is just as complex. The Tyler study is not unusual in failing to indicate with full certainty which therapy is best. The evidence often points to several therapy plans that will "work" and the reasons for their efficacy are hard to sort out. There are at least three ways to deal with such empirical uncertainty.

First, we can go with the **weight of the evidence.** The challenge in this approach is to stay alert for hidden variables and remember that a rose by any other name is still a rose. I recall one study that found no correlation between the parental behavior of asking toddlers to repeat new words and the size of the toddler's vocabularies. However, it turned out that the children who were not being asked to repeat, were natural high imitators who repeated words anyway. This variable had not been included in the initial design so the findings were uninterpretable. Or, as an example of truly obfuscating labels, consider the researcher who compared the effects of HI and LO parental conversation on word learning. It turned out, however, that in the LO conversation condition parents simply read the newspaper—to themselves! We need to get beyond the words and be sure we know exactly who was doing what. With attentive reading, however, a few clear trends do seem to emerge from the empirical literature. For example, a substantial number of studies attest to the efficacy of focused stimulation techniques and I consider this a "best bet" method in language intervention.

A second response to uncertainty turns to **cost-benefit analysis.** Consider, for example, the claim that children with SLI have cognitive processing deficiencies that affect language learning despite their normal-range performance IQ. To evaluate this claim, one would list the consequences of various assumptions paired with true states of affairs (i.e., assuming something to be true when it was not true and when it was true, or assuming something not to be true when it really was true or was not true). There could be costs and benefits at any point in the analysis. For example, a clinician who assumed that children with SLI have cognitive processing deficiencies might test narrative production in a child referred for listening deficits, believing that such deficiencies would have broad consequences. If the assumption were invalid, she might have wasted the time spent in the extra assessment, but if the assumption were true, she would have identified an important area for intervention. Continuing the analysis, if the clinician assumes that children with SLI do *not* have cognitive processing deficiencies but in reality they do, she would miss the child's production problems, and so forth (Johnston, 1999).

And finally, we can be **guided by principle,** selecting the therapy alternative that is most compatible with our theoretical commitments. To my knowledge there is still no research that compares therapy that pursues each goal only until the first signs of knowledge appear and therapy that pursues each goal until considerable mastery is achieved. A language specialist or SLP who is committed to innate language representation and views acquisition as a triggering process might be comfortable with the first criterion. One who believes that language is learned much like everything else, through the application of general cognitive mechanisms, might prefer the second criterion and argue that mastery goals are just as important as initial learning goals.

When all is said and done, there will still be decisions that are difficult to make. In the example of goal attack strategies there is not enough evidence to have any "weight," cost-benefit analysis yields no clear answer, and the very nature of the theoretical issues is hard to discern. We can't wait to decide later because every therapy session and program that we plan must have some sequence of learning goals. One of my students voiced our quandary quite well: "I am struggling with the idea of throwing away instinct about good practice methods, until we have even more data on efficacy. Do you struggle with that as well, or are you comfortable with clinicians limiting their practice to only what is proven effective? I am not sure that I am." Neither am I. At some point, science does end and art begins. But before we decide that we have reached the end of science, let's not forget one further source of efficacy data, namely our own practice. We can at least stay very attentive to a given child's progress and experiment with new approaches whenever language gains are not occurring.❖

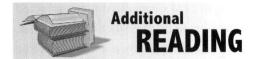

Additional
READING

Leonard, L. (1998). *Children with specific language impairment*. Cambridge, MA: MIT Press. Chapter 10 concerns the nature and efficacy of treatment.

Johnston, J. (1999). Cognitive deficits in specific language impairment: Decision in spite of uncertainty. *Journal of Speech Language Pathology and Audiology, 23*, 65–172.

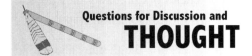

Questions for Discussion and
THOUGHT

1. Here are some additional dimensions of therapy planning that have barely been investigated. Choose one and do a cost-benefit analysis. For each position, list the potential benefits and costs, then decide which one is better. You may place higher value on some cost or benefits than on others.

   • **Criteria for goal completion 40 percent versus 85 percent.** For each criterion level, consider cost and benefit if you use it and it is truly the best choice versus if you use it but it is actually not the best choice.

   • **Use versus non-use of total communication (sign + speech) with *hearing* children.** Consider cost and benefit if you assume that this practice will enhance oral language and in fact it is a hindrance versus if you do not make this assumption and hence do not use the technique but in fact it would have helped. Do you use this procedure? If so, on what grounds?

2. Do you regularly review the research on the efficacy of intervention studies? If not, why not? There are actually very few studies conducted. A yearly review would be sufficient. Discuss how a group of colleagues could manage this task. What resources do you have? Does the local public library have access to journals online (you may be surprised)? Are you near a university? Is there a subscription service you could book (and split the costs)? Is there a student you could hire? Stop your discussion, pick up the phone, or engage the Internet and see if you can answer these questions, then make a plan to share the work of staying current.

Self-Guided Learning
ACTIVITY

Choose one or two children on your caseload who have both phonological and morphological delays. Be sure that the phonological delay is potentially causing difficulty with s/z and d/t either word-final or within clusters. If you find a child who has trouble with both phoneme sets, you can do this exercise using a multiple baseline design and just the one child. If the children have either s/z *or* t/d difficulties, you'll need to compare the progress of two children. Try out Tyler et al.'s (2003) alternating strategy and the strategy of working only on phonology. Assign one method to the past tense and t/d, and the other method to the third person singular present tense and s/z. After one month compare progress. Then, take ten minutes and reflect on this exercise. Was it easy or difficult to conduct? If the latter, what was the source of the difficulty? Could you imagine doing other explicit comparative tests? What methodological issues will you tackle next?

4 Things That Don't Add Up

Computers can figure out all kinds of problems, except for the things in the world that just don't add up.

—James Magary

Assessment protocols emphasize normative, and hence quantitative, judgments. Researchers measure group differences. And, in these days of accountability, we are frequently urged to keep quantitative records of progress. It is easy to start thinking that our goals are measurement goals and that things that are measurable are somehow better, or at least easier to deal with. Inspired by this quotation from the writer James Magary, I want to explore the belief that clinicians and researchers can measure their way out of problems. It turns out that key aspects of both science and practice are not measurable and cannot be quantified. What are these things that just don't add up?

Apples and Fish

The challenge of heterogeneity in clinical research samples is widely acknowledged. Whether it is the autism spectrum, mental retardation, or specific language impairment, the standard diagnostic criteria do not necessarily yield a group of children who have exactly the same developmental profile. Some children with autism evidence global learning delays, others do not. Many English-speaking children with specific language impairments show special difficulty with grammatical morphology but others do not. The essential measurement problem is that apples and fish do not add up—not even as a stew. We can give children the same label, but the differences among them may be more important than the similarities.

Researchers each have their zones of comfort in this matter, depending upon research questions and sampling options, but if they make the wrong decisions the results will be nonsense. Some groups are meant to be heterogeneous—Late Talkers, for example. This label was first applied (and should still be applied) only to children who are evidencing language delays at age 18–24 months. Everyone knew that some of these children were merely starting a bit late and would prove to be perfectly normal learners. However, other children in this group would show persistent difficulties with language learning. The important purpose of the research on Late Talkers was to determine whether, and when, it would be possible to identify children in these two subgroups. (See Essay 10 "Never a Poet" for further discussion of Late Talkers.)

In other instances, heterogeneity in a research group is troublesome. Studies of mental retardation failed for years to acknowledge that children can show global developmental delays for many different reasons, yielding a wide range of behavioral profiles. Persons with Down syndrome, for example, often have motor speech problems but not selective attention deficits, while "rubella babies" tend to have just the opposite profile. Studies of retardation that ignored such differences could be very misleading.

As research consumers, we need to pay careful attention to the criteria that are used to select participants in a study and decide whether they are appropriate for the purposes of the research. For example, if the researchers are evaluating the general language outcomes from a parent education program, the degree of dissimilarity among the children may be irrelevant. Parent education sessions for early intervention are, and are meant to be, generically applied to all children with language learning difficulties. On the other hand, if the researchers are studying causal factors (e.g., the role of social knowledge in the pragmatic deficits associated with autism) it will be important to acknowledge that children diagnosed as autistic can have very different sorts of social-emotional profiles. Some avoid social contact, others welcome it. Treating autistic persons as though they all had the same problems may result in confusion rather than clarity.

Alphas

If you have ever taken a course in statistics, you may have noticed that p and q add up, but alpha does not. Alpha levels are not statistical outcomes that are calculated. They are arbitrary points along a continuum of risk that are selected by the researcher following an analysis of the likely costs of being wrong. When they use an alpha level of .05, for example, researchers have decided that if p—the probability of getting a result on the basis of chance alone—is greater than 5 times in 100, the risk and costs of being wrong are too great and they will therefore not treat the finding as valid. Alpha judgments are crucial since they affect the interpretation of findings and, ultimately, the likelihood that a line of investigation will be continued. Setting an alpha level at .01 may mean that an effect worth studying will be set aside as a chance result, but it could also prevent future research dollars being wasted. On the other hand, setting an alpha level at .1 may call attention to true differences that would otherwise be ignored. Researchers need to weigh the costs and benefits and consider the entire body of evidence to date as they make these decisions.

Clinicians face a similar challenge in establishing the line between normalcy and disorder, and these decisions are likewise important since they determine which children will receive support and service. Although alpha levels and the boundaries of disorder could in principle be supported by mathematical modeling, the state of our current understanding does not permit a quantitative approach.

The traditional alpha level in behavioral research is .05, but this value is entirely arbitrary. As we read studies that report "nonsignificant" findings and provide the actual probabilities (e.g., $p = .072$), we may decide for ourselves that a "nonsignificant" finding in the range between $p = .05$ and $p = .10$ is in fact something we want to explore anyway, especially in the cases where there is little cost if it were untrue and good payoff if it were true. Similarly, in current SLP practice, the boundary line for disorder is typically set at -1.5 *SD* or -1 *SD*, essentially the 10th to the 15th percentile. There is to my knowledge, no empirical justification for this cutoff, and over the last 30 years it has drifted upward from -2 *SD* to -1.5 *SD* and even -1 *SD*. Some of the reasons for this change are relatively positive, for example, the increased availability of service and a desire to assist those children who could perform at age level with only a moderate level of help. Other reasons for the change are more questionable, for example, difficulty in finding seriously delayed children in a given locale to participate in research studies.

Eventually we may learn that children who function at the -1.5 *SD* level are categorically different than children with lesser problems. But in the meantime, decisions about which child has a language impairment cannot be made on the basis of measurement alone. As clinicians, we would be wise to let the boundary of disorder be permeable. If we treat this arbitrary number as somehow "given," we run the risk of underestimating, or overestimating, the personal and social significance of a given child's language delay.

Trunks, Legs, and Tails

I allude here, of course, to the familiar story of the blind men and the elephant. There are two senses in which the elephant's parts do not add up. First, each of the blind men considered his particular part of the elephant to be the whole and hence came to a wrong conclusion. We have done the same thing. In the late 1970s, researchers said that the language development of children with SLI followed normal patterns and clinicians argued the opposite. It turned out that each of us was treating a part of the picture as if it were the whole. Studies ultimately revealed essential normalcy within each linguistic domain, but asynchrony in rates of development from one domain to the next.

As a second example, think about the initial studies of parent education programs in early language intervention. Researchers at first failed to demonstrate language change in the children and so concluded that the programs had not been effective. *Parents* had changed in their attitudes and practices toward their children, but the significance of this finding was discounted. However, studies showing that parent-child interactions clearly affect patterns of language learning (Hart & Risley, 1995) and progress in therapy (Schery, 1985) suggest that parental change should be treated as a legitimate, if incomplete, index of program efficacy.

In these examples, a part was mistaken for a whole, leading researchers and clinicians to the wrong conclusion. As clinical consumers of the research literature, we need to remember that researchers can only describe what they look at. There is important selectivity in every data set. As we read research reports we need to step back a moment and think about the questions that were not asked and the observations that were not made. For example, the first research studies attesting to the effectiveness of Fast ForWord® used test scores rather than looked at everyday, functional communication (Tallal et al., 1996). If these researchers had looked at children's actual communication patterns, they might have come to a different conclusion.

Good clinical practice likewise requires systematic investigation of all of the parts. It is very easy, for example, when evaluating a language sample, to look for grammatical errors and, finding none, conclude that the child has no language problem. However, if we were to look at a different part of the elephant, such as the proportion of complex utterances in the child's speech, we might come to the opposite conclusion. Checklists can help us maintain a broad vision.

An even greater challenge lies in the fact that elephants are more than a collection of trunks and legs and tails. Collections of parts lack integrative structure and coherence. Structures such as part-whole relationship or causal dependency are not easily measured, but are crucial aspects of the whole. To understand how the parts relate to each other we again need theory. Let's think further about language samples. Analysis with standardized scoring systems or with Systematic

Thinking About Child Language

Analysis of Language Transcripts (SALT; Miller & Iglesias, 2003–2005) can provide us with a list of parts, but language is a system, not a collection. Certain sentence types may be missing from the child's language because the auxiliary class is not yet present; a child may lack clear reference because of word finding difficulties; or, a child may have surprising lexical strengths because he or she has advanced nonverbal concepts despite grammatical delays. These statements are all about the connections between the parts of an integrated language system. They are challenging to understand, but crucial to good educational planning.

Personal Values, Social Trends, Political Will, Economic Factors, Research Goals and Paths

Finally, let's reflect on the choices we make about the focus of research or of clinical practice. What questions are worth studying? What problems are worth remediating? However difficult it may be, we evaluate our research and clinical priorities and choose the questions and programs that are important. To do so, we must think

about personal values, political currents, technology, and the state of the art on any given research topic or clinical practice. Most of this cannot be measured.

As an interesting case in point, consider the research on SLI and grammatical morphology. This work has been some of the most programmatic and theory-driven research in our field. We began by discovering the special vulnerability of the domain, then we identified it as being language-specific, and eventually explained slow learning and poor performance on grammatical morphemes by appeal to faulty representation or processing constraints. The studies continue, but

it seems to me that the theoretical positions have ossified of late, and momentum has slowed. Perhaps it is time to move on to some of the topics that we are not yet studying:

- When and for whom do particular intervention procedures work best? Are parent education programs equally effective with syntactic and lexical goals, and with Stage 4 as well as Stage 2 children?

- What is the role of culture in treating and understanding language disorders? Should we allow cultural values to determine program goals and methods? Whose culture?

- What are the long-term economic costs and savings of early language intervention? We desperately need to assess the current data, figure out which pieces are missing, and build the models that will increase our clout at the public policy table.

I'm sure you could add to the list. The point here is not the contents of the list, but the fact of the list and the choices it implies. Researchers want to make a difference and we need good measurement to reach this goal, but to find the key topics we must consider not only the data, but personal values, social trends, political will, economic factors, and the goals and paths of past investigators.

The clinical parallels are quite clear. In these days of limited resources, every SLP faces hard decisions about service priorities and programs. Should we continue to provide home-based service if center-based service is more efficient? Should we develop a parent education program for disadvantaged families; a preschool program that integrates typical and disordered learners; or a clinical education program for young professionals? Should we see fewer children more often? And if so, which ones? The list is endless. The really important fact to acknowledge is that the answers to these questions are not out there already, waiting to be found. These questions must be answered by individual SLPs or service teams, after careful consideration of values and commitments, as well as local circumstances and options.

In short, measurement, while important, will not solve many of our most important research and clinical challenges. In addition to new research tools or new clinical assessment and intervention procedures, we need imagination, rigor, flexibility, good sense, and good theory. We also need the courage to make hard decisions and the discipline to stay informed.❖

NOTE: This essay is an expanded version of an invited lecture presented at the Madison Symposium for Research in Child Language Disorders, University of Wisconsin, Madison, June, 2003.

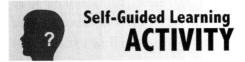

Questions for Discussion and
THOUGHT

1. Isn't it ultimately possible to measure anything? Are the examples in this essay truly instances of areas that can't be measured, or is it just that no one has done so yet? If at least some of the areas discussed here could be quantified, would it be a good idea to do so?

2. If all of the scientists decide to set their alpha levels at .05, why should we decide any differently?

3. Reflect on your work over the last week, both as individuals and as a group. Try to identify actions that were driven by personal values or economic factors rather than (or as well as) empirical facts.

Self-Guided Learning
ACTIVITY

Choose a child (or two) on your caseload for whom you have standardized scores for phonology, vocabulary, and syntax. (This could be a SALT *z*-score, or a subtest score from the TOLD or CELF). If at all possible, use vocabulary and syntax scores from the same mode (i.e., both comprehension or both production). Now consider the scores as a profile of integrated language abilities and make a list of the influences from one domain to the other. Is there anything about this child's phonology that constrains or facilitates morphology? Does vocabulary constrain or facilitate syntax? And so on. If you find a likely zone of connection between two domains, plan a therapy task that addresses or takes advantage of this fact.

Language Disorders in Children

T he first conference on a condition known as "childhood aphasia" was held at Stanford University in 1960. Forty-five years later, the name has changed to "specific language impairment" (SLI), but the nature of the condition remains a puzzle. Language is, after all, a product of the mind. If it doesn't develop on the predicted course, some mental function must be implicated. Moreover, we know that language is one of the most important human tools for reasoning and learning. Children who do not use language efficiently and reliably should have some intellectual disadvantage. How could it be possible for children to be normally developing in every respect except language?

The essays in this section concern our continuing investigations into questions related to the nature of SLI. Is memory involved? How can you be smart without good language skills? Is this really a single condition? What happens to kids who start out as poor language learners? In answering these questions about SLI, however, we also learn something about memory, utterance production, IQ tests, and other areas that will help us think more clearly about all the children we serve.

5 Pitfalls and Promises in the Study of SLI

Why Study Specific Language Impairment?

I have been studying children with specific language impairments (SLI) for almost 40 years—essentially from the time they were invented. Children in this diagnostic group are defined by a developmental dissociation between language and other aspects of cognition, with language skills markedly lagging behind other areas of learning. As a young clinician, I was intrigued by SLI as a window to thought that was not yet shaped by language, or perhaps as a demonstration that human intellect could prevail in silence. However, these early interests soon evolved into a less romantic agenda. The overarching goal of this agenda was to delineate and understand the relationships that might exist between language and nonverbal cognition. These relationships, as I came to understand them, included:

- Language as the product of general information processing mechanisms

- Language as the representation of the child's conceptual or world knowledge

- Language as a necessary tool for intellectual growth

Since children with SLI offered an opportunity to explore each of these relations, research with these children could not only help us understand the nature of language impairment, but also the general nature of language and intellectual development in all children.

The basic rationale for the research program was that each of the possible relationships between language and nonverbal cognition could be disconfirmed by data from children with SLI. For example:

- If children with SLI turned out to have intact processing mechanisms, it would call into question the idea that language is the product of general cognitive information systems.

- If children with SLI did not express meanings that were, like their nonverbal cognition, more advanced than their language level, the claim that language represents the child's available concepts would be constrained.

33

- If children with SLI showed age-level conceptual and reasoning achievements despite their language delays, we would need to qualify the claim that language is integral to intellectual growth.

The Story Thus Far

Over a number of years now, my student colleagues and I have observed children with SLI performing on a wide range of reasoning, processing, and language tasks. Instead of intact cognitive processes, we found children who were challenged by the resource demands of ordinal relations (Johnston & Smith, 1989), were slow in manipulating visual images (Johnston & Ellis Weismer, 1983), and had difficulties with cross-modal perception (Kamhi, 1981). Instead of seeing content in advance of form, we saw six-year-olds with delays in narrative coherence (Oxelgren, 1998; Oxelgren & Johnston, 1996), and use of mental state predicates that resembled that of language peers rather than age peers (Johnston et al., 2001). Instead of conceptual and reasoning advances, we found two-year delays in conservation reasoning that was tested nonverbally (Johnston & Ramstad, 1983), and a negative correlation between cognitive efficiency and the use of problem-solving language (Sturn & Johnston, 1999).

We did find some evidence of the expected dissociation between language and nonverbal cognition. For example, five-year-old children with SLI did achieve age-appropriate success on spatial reasoning tasks, albeit through trial and error, and preschool children with SLI used communication predicates such as *say* and *show* at earlier than expected language levels. But these signs of dissociation always emerged as secondary analyses in studies where the major findings pointed in another direction.

As results accumulated from our lab and elsewhere, I became more and more convinced that SLI isn't really very specific, or for that matter, essentially linguistic. Language development in these children was perhaps lagging behind other aspects of cognitive development, but the gaps were often quite modest and there was much evidence of mutual connection and influence. It was ultimately the association, not the dissociation that was compelling. Rather than disconfirm, the evidence from children with SLI actually provides additional evidence that:

- General cognitive processing mechanisms contribute to language learning.

- Language form or experience can limit meanings.

- Language is a major contributor to intellectual development.

This picture of association between language and cognition brings a new set of reasons to study children with SLI—to identify the ways in which language serves thought. One important language function is to code experience and the interim products of thought so that these can be incorporated into more complex chains of reasoning. Studies of verbal and nonverbal working memory and of memory strategies in children with SLI will help us understand these processes and also the potential costs of poor language proficiency.

The Pitfalls of SLI in Research and Clinical Practice

The research opportunities presented by children with SLI are accompanied by equally potent challenges—the pitfalls that come with the promises. Two of the most fundamental challenges come from the notion of nonverbal IQ, and from the fact that SLI is underspecified.

Nonverbal IQ

All IQ tests are nothing more or less than a set of intellectual tasks. Nonverbal (or performance) IQ is established by performance on one set of tasks, and the nature of these tasks will influence the test outcome. Nonverbal intelligence is no more monolithic than verbal intelligence. In the same way we talk about vocabulary knowledge, grammar, phonology, and language use, we can talk about memory, attention, perception, inferential reasoning, conceptual schemes, and world knowledge. Any nonverbal IQ test measures only a subset of these structures and functions. That is why it is possible to take a group of children and say that they have normal nonverbal IQ and also that they are two years delayed in conservation reasoning. The fact that children with SLI have normal-range performance IQ is not trivial, but we should not assume that a score derived from a perceptual matching task gives us information about memory or conceptual development.

Task analysis of various performance IQ scales is an important first step in understanding the nonverbal status of a group of SLI children, but even that information can be misleading. Some years ago (Johnston, 1982a) I analyzed the item content of the Leiter International Performance Scale (now replaced by a later version) and found that below the age of 7 or so there was a preponderance of perceptual items (i.e., items that could be solved simply by noting the physical characteristics of the objects such as color or shape). I hypothesized that SLI children were earning their IQ points on these items rather than on the more conceptually

35

demanding items such as those that require the child to see the similarity of three dots and three lines. It turned out that children in both groups did relatively better on the perceptual items. This of course means that the scope of the test items and the scope of the IQ were not actually equivalent. Although the test items included many with a conceptual content, children from 3 to 6 years of age do poorly on those items and the resulting IQ primarily reflects perceptual abilities.

Underspecification

Although exclusionary criteria for the diagnosis of SLI seem quite rigorous, there is much that is left open. The area(s) of language that are affected, the magnitude of the delay, the presence of social problems, the relative strength of visual imagery, the developmental level of the child, and many other important areas of function can all vary widely among children who otherwise qualify as SLI. This lack of specificity causes problems of two sorts.

The first problem arises directly from the developmental differences just described—and that is the problem of **heterogeneity.** Much of the research on SLI draws its conclusions from the performance patterns of groups of children taken as a whole. I recently became curious about how many individual children in our research samples actually conform to the general trends, so I reviewed five sets of language data archived in my lab. Three of them, involving 42 preschoolers with SLI, included analyses of grammatical morphology and variables such as percentage occurrence in obligatory contexts. In each of these studies, the SLI group did, indeed, use grammatical morphemes less well on average than would be expected for either their age or language level. But it was also true that a goodly number of those in each study, 30 to 40 percent, failed to show this pattern. Diversity was also seen in two sets of narrative data, from 53 school-age children with SLI. When we looked at the relative strength of story content and grammaticality, children with SLI showed two quite different patterns. The majority told adequate to strong stories riddled with grammatical error, but some 35 percent of the children told stories that were fully grammatical, albeit dull and/or incoherent (Johnston, 2005b).

The challenges of heterogeneity grow larger as sample sizes get smaller, but researchers at least have some coping strategies. To insure that readers and other scientists can draw conclusions across studies, we provide the widest possible range of descriptive data about the children we study. For example, even when receptive language abilities are not used as a criterion for SLI or are not the focus of a given project, we report receptive language scores. This allows researchers who do have an interest in receptive language to make use of our findings.

The more serious problem with underspecification is the hidden companion to heterogeneity—**selectivity.** Unless we have funding for epidemiological studies, most of the children with SLI who participate in research will be referred by clinics and schools. This means that some professional, usually a speech-language pathologist, has initially decided that these children have a language problem. Since a wide range of language problems will identify a child as having SLI, there is ample room for what I call *diagnostic dialects.* Different therapists with different educational backgrounds, interests, and abilities will emphasize different aspects of language in their diagnostic decisions, and will prioritize their caseloads in different ways. The consequences of these clinical decisions are quite evident in the research literature where it would seem at first that all the SLI children in British Columbia live in the region of Salmon Arm, or that all the children with semantic-pragmatic impairments live on the North American East Coast and Great Britain. Actually, these distributional facts are more likely to reflect the diagnostic interests and priorities of particular professional communities. I think we have underestimated the consequences of these diagnostic biases, and a practical solution has yet to emerge. At the least, we will need better communication between the clinical and research communities, and an ongoing commitment to continuing professional education by both.

Pitfalls and Promises in Clinical Practice

Given all the factors that determine language growth (see Essay 1), it would not surprise me to learn that children with SLI have problems with language learning for a variety of reasons. We'll set aside the theorizing for the moment, however, and concentrate on the practical ramifications of what children with SLI have taught us about cognition and language, and about diversity.

First, although as SLPs we are most comfortable with assessing and teaching communication skills, the research summarized above indicates that we will rarely meet a child who "only has language problems." Language is the product of the highly evolved human mind and when it doesn't emerge on track, something is seriously wrong. Likewise, language is the tool of intellect and when this tool is not available, children will be hindered in complex problem-solving tasks. Viewed from this perspective, language disorders always point to impairments elsewhere, such as in processing or in reasoning.

Second, clinicians need to become more familiar with the tests used to establish performance (i.e., nonverbal) IQ so that we know whether a given test taps into perception, classification, memory, or some other functional property of cognition. The Buros Institute's *Mental Measurements Yearbooks* (Buros Institute, 1938–2005; per-item purchase available online, www.unl.edu/buros) are an invaluable resource for information about the structure, tasks, and reliability of many cognitive tests.

Third, the differences found within research samples of SLI children invite us to think more comprehensively about what constitutes a language problem. I want to spend a bit more time on this idea. We all have our own beliefs about which aspects of language knowledge and use are most important in the evaluation of everyday communication, and the assessment tools we know best are the ones that test our favorite parts of language. But sometimes, we need to look elsewhere. For me, the biggest steps came with the advent of developmental pragmatics.

I started paying attention to pragmatics (i.e., language in context) when I was a student at the University of California–Berkeley, and Elizabeth Bates came to our department as a visiting faculty member. I was busy writing my dissertation on the connections between lexical development and spatial conceptualization, and I wasn't enthusiastic about expanding my horizons. Semantics and syntax were enough. Then one evening Liz and I had dinner together, and in the course of the conversation I realized that if I were to remain a responsible clinician, I could no longer ignore pragmatics. It wasn't enough to describe the language forms in a child's repertoire. I also needed to pay attention to whether the child could use those familiar forms appropriately and reliably in the service of particular communication acts. Ultimately that realization led me to a totally new, more functional understanding of grammar and of the communicative cost of language impairments. I still look first at morphosyntax and vocabulary when I assess children's language, but now I also try to evaluate patterns of use.

Some of you may share my biases, others of you may focus more naturally on communicative success. If so, your challenge is to consciously remember that some children fail to communicate only because they lack knowledge of the requisite language forms. This is particularly seen in children who seem to be having trouble with topic maintenance. I recently reviewed a conversational transcript from C.J., a seven-year-old with fragile X syndrome, who frequently made the following sort of conversational error:

SLP: Why is he going to work?

C.J.: Gonna sit now.

At first C.J. seems to be ignoring the question and pursuing her own play routine. But after reviewing the entire transcript, I think that C.J. just doesn't understand "Why" and has difficulty with the spatial meaning of "going to." She answers the question as if it were "What is he gonna do?" This child has a definite language problem, but I doubt it will be remedied by focusing on whether or not she responds to questions. Once she knows the necessary language, her conversational responsiveness should improve.

In sum, the diagnostic criteria for SLI underspecify the condition. Children who are diagnosed with SLI can—at least in principle—have delays or difficulties with any one or more of the domains of language: phonology, relational semantics, lexical semantics, syntax, morphology, and pragmatics. This means that the training, abilities, and interests of a given SLP can easily lead her or him to emphasize one type of language problem and ignore others. Service policies and the availability of funding probably play a role in these decisions as well. Whatever the source of our assessment biases, we need to override them and be as thorough as possible in our observation of a child's language and communication patterns. A broader range of information will help us prioritize therapy goals, think more clearly about connections between the various aspects of language, and make better referrals to research projects.❖

NOTE: An earlier version of this essay was presented at the July 2002 Congress of the International Association for the Study of Child Language, Madison, WI.

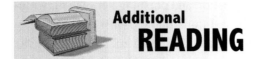

Additional
READING

Johnston, J. (1982a). Interpreting the Leiter IQ: Performance Profiles of Young Normal and Language Disordered Children. *Journal of Speech and Hearing Research, 25,* 291–296.

Simons, H. (1996). The paradox of case study. *Cambridge Journal of Education, 26,* 225–240.

NOTE: Case-based research can provide an effective foil for the underspecified group study; moreover, it is one way that clinicians can make important contributions to intervention research.

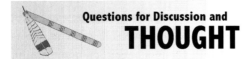

Questions for Discussion and
THOUGHT

1. Select and obtain a nonverbal intelligence test that can be used by an SLP, e.g., Columbia Mental Maturity Scale (CMMS), Leiter International Performance Scale (LIPS), Ravens Progressive Matrices (Ravens), or Test of Nonverbal Intelligence (TONI). Discuss the items and subscales of the test. What is, and is not, being measured?

2. What would be the costs and benefits of providing intervention to a child whose communication problems were different than the sort you usually see?

3. If you don't routinely obtain nonverbal IQ scores (either from your own testing or from the psychologist down the hall), what would be the costs and benefits of doing so?

4. Consider your group's involvement in collaborative research. Under what circumstances are you willing to find participants for researchers? What are your concerns about research, if any? What time of year is best? Would you be able to do any assessments for the research team? What are your agency's or your district's policies about participating in research?

Self-Guided Learning
ACTIVITIES

1. The answers to the questions in discussion question 4 would be of great interest to researchers at the nearest university Communication Sciences and Disorders program. Think about a summary letter you could send or a phone number you could use to start the ball rolling.

2. Borrow or purchase a nonverbal intelligence test (see question 1) and administer it to two of your clients—one you are sure is "bright," the other to a child whose intellectual abilities are in question. Observe the differences in task performance. (Do not record or report the scores, since some experience is needed first to insure their validity.)

6 The Morphology Gene

I will never forget the Madison Symposium at which Myrna Gopnik announced that she and her colleagues had evidence of the morphology gene. The data concerned a British family that for generations had manifested serious language problems. Attributing their problems to genetic endowment seemed so tidy…and so final.

We now know that members of this particular family have pervasive cognitive and speech problems as well as language problems and hence cannot stand as proof of a specific, genetically based deficit in grammar. The idea of a morphology gene nevertheless remains intriguing. If language abilities are part of our human endowment, could we indeed be hard-wired for morphology? How would that work? Genetic researchers have recently tackled everything from potatoes to Parkinson's, so genetic studies of language impairment should not come as a surprise. Here is a sampling.

Family Aggregation Studies

In one set of studies, researchers have identified children with language impairment and then looked to see whether other members of the family have histories of speech, language, or reading difficulties. Recently, Tallal et al. (2001) went beyond history taking and actually tested family members to ascertain their current level of language function. The targeted group, or "probands" in the parlance of genetic studies, were 22 school-age children with normal-range nonverbal IQ and TOLD/TOAL scores below 85 (or the average of TOLD/TOAL + TTFC below 85). An age-matched control group was also selected. Parents and siblings of children in the SLI and the control group were then given the TOLD/TOAL and TTFC. Some 31 percent of the family members related to the SLI children, but only 7 percent of the family members related to the control children showed current language deficits. Mothers and fathers were equally likely to have language impairment (28 versus 31 percent), but brothers were more likely than sisters to be impaired (44 versus 15 percent).

Twin Studies

Investigators have also used groups of twins to measure the degree to which language abilities are genetically determined. In this approach, pairs of *identical* twins (MZ, monozygotic—a single ovum split during development) are compared to pairs of *fraternal* twins (DZ, dizygotic—two ova). Typically, one member of each twin pair has been previously diagnosed as language impaired. Language scores are then obtained and used to determine whether the twin pair is *concordant*, that is, shares the same trait (i.e., language impairment). If language disorders are genetically determined, the MZ twins should show higher rates of concordance than the DZ twins. Combining the findings from five recent studies, Stromswold (2001) reports a concordance rate of 84 percent for MZ twin pairs and 50 percent for DZ twin pairs—a difference that is statistically reliable and points to the definite presence of genetic factors.

Language researchers with twin data often go beyond rates of concordance and estimate the strength of the genetic factors by calculating the correlation between the test scores earned by the two members of the pair. Findings vary considerably from study to study depending on age, language domain, and test, but they consistently point to major genetic components in the language performance of children with SLI. For example, Bishop et al. (1995) report MZ test correlations in the order of .7 to .8 and DZ test correlations in the order of .2 to .4, yielding a *heritability* estimate of about 1.0. That is, virtually all of the differences among their school-age children with SLI could be attributed to genetic factors. In another recent twin study (Dale et al., 1998), the group differences heritability indicated that 73 percent of the variance among two-year-olds with language delay was due to genetic factors, and only 18 percent due to shared environment.

What Does "Genetic" Mean?

These are impressive studies (one of the twin studies has more than 3000 pairs!), and the findings are dramatic, but they are really just a beginning. Knowing that there *is* a genetic influence is far different than understanding the nature of that influence. As Bruce Tomblin noted in a discussion session at that same Madison Symposium, we still must find out if there is one affected gene, or several; if the effect is dominant or recessive; which physical mechanisms are affected; and how these effects impinge on language learning.

Mode of Transmission

Full answers to these questions will require different sorts of research methods including actual DNA analysis, but there are hints in the aggregation data. Stromswold (2001) observes that the rates of family member involvement don't fit any of the classic inheritance models very well (e.g., autosomal dominant, autosomal recessive). Autosomal dominant transmission, for example, would cause most probands to have just one affected parent, but in fact only 32 percent of them do. She concludes that whatever the genetic mode of transmission may be, it is not likely that there is only one affected gene. Either there are several different transmission modes, each operating in some proportion of cases, or there are a number of different genes that act in concert to create the language difficulties.

This Is the Morphology Gene?

Researchers are now beginning to report DNA analyses of affected and unaffected members of families that show an aggregation of SLI. So far some eight chromosomal sites have emerged as potentially relevant, including 7q31, 6p21, 15q21, and 13q21 (Bartlett et al., 2002). Interestingly, these sites have also emerged in studies of reading, Tourette's, autism, and AD/HD. They are sites known to be associated with the gamma-aminobutyric-acid beta-receptor, a major inhibitory neurotransmitter, and with fatty acid and membrane phospholipid metabolism, among others. What this has to do with grammatical morphology is, of course, still quite unclear.

Implications for Practice

The moral to this story is that when you go looking for the morphology gene you may end up with a fatty acid metabolism gene. And then what? Until we know how to get from fatty acids to grammatical morphology, the fact that SLI has a genetic basis is not particularly useful information. In order to make use of genetic research in intervention, we need to know more about the physical consequences of the gene abnormality, and the implications of those physical facts for psychological functioning. Moreover, since there is considerable agreement that language abilities are the result of many genes, each with a relatively small effect, acting together and in combination with environmental factors (e.g., Plomin & Dale, 2000), we will need to know about many causal chains. When genetic research begins to provide this sort of information, we may discover that the genetically caused impediments to language learning are old friends, such as rate of processing and auditory memory span.

Whatever the outcome, the genetic research on SLI is not likely to be either tidy or final. As Annette Karmiloff-Smith, current Director of the Neurocognitive Development Unit at London's Institute of Child Health sees it, "There is no simple one-to-one mapping between genes and cognitive outcomes, so the story is going to be exceedingly complex" (Serratrice, 2005, p.7).

There *is* one area of practice that is affected by our knowledge that specific language impairments in childhood may be genetically determined, namely, the explanations and advice we give to family members. I see two major implications. First, extended descriptions of communication and syntax skills may exceed the metalinguistic abilities of at least one third of the parents of SLI children. They may not be aware of their child's language limitations, or may not be able to understand your language analyses. Even if they desire to participate in the intervention process, family members who themselves have language limitations may be unable to consciously provide examples of anything other than simple vocabulary goals. We should be careful not to interpret their lack of success as a lack of cooperation or caring. Better still, we could avoid such disappointments by listening carefully to parental language before we assign tasks that require higher level language skills, and by having alternative sorts of home programs at the ready.

Second, parents want to understand the nature of their children's communication or academic difficulties. They may be relieved to learn that these difficulties are not due to poor parenting. Moreover, learning that language impairments are likely to be genetic in origin and "run in families" may lead them to identify other family members who have had language-related learning problems. As we share our confidence in their child's ability to learn and achieve, we may actually help them view their own, their spouse's, or their other children's abilities in a more positive light. As we point to the visual strengths, social intuitions, or native intelligence of children with SLI, we may be giving family members the tools to appreciate their own competencies. ❖

Thinking About Child Language

Questions for Discussion and
THOUGHT

1. What are the potential problems that could arise if you explain to a parent that specific language difficulties often run in families?

2. Would you alter your treatment planning if you knew for sure that a child's language difficulties were genetic, and if so, how?

3. What symptoms of low language proficiency could be evident in a parent's language? How would you change the way you talk about a child's language difficulty if the parents seemed to have language problems?

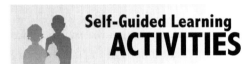

Self-Guided Learning
ACTIVITIES

1. If you work in a setting where you do regular intake assessments of young children, add this question to your interview: "Are there other members of your family who were late talkers or were slow in learning to read?" After the next 10 or 20 assessments, tally the number of parents who said yes. Did your percentages correspond with the research reviewed above? Why or why not?

2. Review your current caseload, and identify the 1 to 2 children who are most likely to have genetically based language disorders. (Look for children with serious delays that seem quite specific to language.) Have they been making good progress in treatment? What does this imply?

7 Difficulties with Language Formulation

Types of Developmental Language Disorder

For decades, researchers have tried to come up with a scheme for classifying sub-groups of children with developmental language disorders. Some have focused on the presumed cause of the disorder, such as autism, deafness, or developmental delay. Others have focused on the areas of language that seemed most affected and have proposed categories such as semantic-pragmatic disorder or grammatical-SLI. Still others have grouped children according to whether their language difficulties are observable only in expressive language, or in language comprehension as well.

The clinical utility of these taxonomies has been disappointing. There are as yet no treatments that are specific to a particular etiology, and labels such as "semantic-pragmatic disorder" merely summarize the results of routine language profiling. There is some evidence that children with "receptive" language problems have a poorer prognosis (Bishop & Edmundson, 1987), but this realization hasn't generated new treatment strategies.

The one distinction that seems to have real clinical promise is the distinction between *knowing* a language pattern, and *using* that pattern easily and reliably in everyday speech. This is, of course, the very old distinction between competence and performance, a distinction that remains useful even though the boundary between *knowing* and *using* can become quite fuzzy. Despite the familiarity of these notions, we often miss their full range of application. We are sensitive to performance difficulties in the comprehension of utterances (often referred to as auditory processing problems), but we often forget the reality of performance difficulties in the *production* of utterances.

Children with Language Performance Problems

Current models of speech production (e.g., Bock & Levelt, 1994) envision a system in which many independent mental modules work in a coordinated, often simultaneous manner to generate an utterance. Rather than completing all of the grammatical coding before proceeding to the phonological coding, or all of the phonological coding before initiating articulation, it seems that our production system sends each product down the line as soon as it is ready. This means that we may be articulating the first part of an utterance while we are still looking for the words that will express the final part of our idea. Viewed this way, speech processes are incremental in that they function on successive pieces of utterances. It is easy to see how such a system could break down. Anything that slows the processing of a given increment (e.g., problems finding a word or implementing a new syntactic pattern), will affect downstream increments that are waiting for it. The result can be a visible moment of disruption: a pause, a reformulation, a self-repetition, or even the loss of the final elements in the utterance.

Some speakers seem particularly vulnerable to this sort of speech error. The Reverend William Archibald Spooner, for example, was famous for mixing sounds in words and producing phrases such as "a blushing crow" (crushing blow). More to the point here, however, are the findings of Miller (1987) and Fletcher (1992), who each found groups of children who were best characterized as having performance difficulties with language production. Miller's data, for example, indicated three such groups, characterized by either sentence formulation problems, word finding problems, or rate and fluency problems. Fletcher's data likewise revealed children who had "structure building problems…and were very prone to error on-line" (p. 161). A recent study of normally developing children helps us put these findings in perspective.

Sentence Disruptions in the Development of Grammar

Rispoli and Hadley (2001) analyzed spontaneous language samples from 26 children aged 2;6 to 4, taped while interacting with their caregiver. They took all of the intelligible, active, declarative sentences in these samples—some 17,000 utterances—and divided them into those that contained disruptions and those that did not. Disruptions included any obvious break in the steady production of the sentence (i.e., nonemphatic repetitions, fillers such as *um*, silent pauses, and revisions of all sorts). Rispoli and Hadley then did a number of developmental analyses to see what factors were correlated with the incidence of these disruptions. The findings that really caught my attention were these:

- The rate of disruption did not correlate with age or developmental level.

- As MLU increased, there was an increasing difference between the length of utterances with and without disruptions.

The first finding indicates that production difficulties can occur at all language levels and have more to do with speaker characteristics than with the challenges of any particular language target. The second finding implies that disruptions tend to occur on the longest and most complex sentences of a given child. Rispoli and Hadley call these sentences "the leading edge" of the child's competence and note that "the demands of such sentences exceed the child's ability to produce a sentence in a smooth, graceful manner...The structures in leading-edge sentences have already emerged. Children will attempt [them] because they lie within their range of competence" (p. 1142), but since some of the required processing modules are new or newly organized, children may not succeed in producing these sentences without disruption.

Implications for Practice

These findings point to an important conclusion: language development is more than the *acquisition* of words, grammatical patterns, social rules of usage, narrative schemes, and so on. Language development also entails the *increasing control* of this knowledge. Child speakers at all language levels will have some forms that are very familiar, often used, and easy to produce. Other forms will not yet have reached this level of control and will be the points at which production breakdowns can occur.

Rispoli and Hadley's (2001) work makes it clear that production breakdowns are not necessarily a symptom of disorder. They occur quite normally for some children throughout the course of development. It remains possible that the children identified by Miller (1987) or Fletcher (1992) showed some abnormal patterns of disruption. Perhaps disruptions occurred on early—as well as later—learned forms or occurred at unusual positions in the sentence. One study does suggest that further research on error patterns would be valuable. Namazi (1999; Namazi & Johnston, 1997), found that preschoolers with SLI were more prone to omit grammatical morphemes in sentences with greater syntactic complexity, and that this was not true for younger, language-matched peers.

Even if they turn out to be developmentally appropriate, disruptions in language production invite intervention. The six-year-old who has just learned to expand the verb phrase with modal auxiliaries is delayed in the acquisition of that form—and is also delayed in its mastery. Many of the children on our caseloads, especially those of elementary school age, are still having production difficulties with complex sentences, even when they "know" the requisite words and patterns. These children do not need assistance in acquiring new language knowledge, they need assistance in mastering the language they know. Unfortunately, the intervention literature seldom addresses this need.

One of the best articles on mastery learning was published some years ago by Culatta and Horn (1982). Given the theoretical views of that time, they describe their program as being designed to aid "generalization of grammatical rules to spontaneous discourse" (p. 174). From our perspective now, what they were doing was helping children automatize (i.e., master) grammatical patterns. Their basic strategy was to provide opportunities for children to repeatedly use sentence patterns and morphological forms that they already knew, in communicative contexts that became more and more demanding. At the start of the program, two potential targets were selected for each child (e.g., copula and embedded *not*). All targets were forms that the child used with 100 percent reliability in structured therapy tasks, but with only 30 to 70 percent reliability in spontaneous speech. The authors then created role-playing activities that invited use of these forms (e.g., having the child describe store products to customers, "This is good soap. It is soap for clothes"). As the sessions evolved, the communication tasks became more difficult (e.g., describing goods to a stock boy *and* telling him where to put them). At the same time that the communication contexts became less focused on the target, the clinician also used fewer examples of the target form in her own speech. Language samples taken during the course of therapy demonstrated that children became consistent in the use of the target forms as therapy was provided, and target form use was still consistent one month later.

Developmental research on disruptions in language production implies that some of the children on our caseloads need performance goals as well as knowledge goals. The child who has just learned the past tense -*ed*, or even the child who uses -*ed* 100 percent of the time in a structured communication game, may not be able to readily produce this form on the playground. Traditionally this has been viewed as a problem in generalization, but I think it is better understood as a lack of automaticity or control. Cullatta and Horn (1982) make it clear that it is possible to move children along the road to mastery by gradually and systematically removing the discourse supports that we originally provide to help them acquire a new form. Now we need to identify the children and the forms for which such treatment is warranted.❖

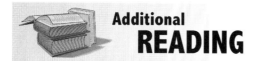

Additional
READING

Bock, K., & Levelt, W. (1994). Language production: Grammatical encoding. In M. A. Gernsbacher (Ed.), *Handbook of psycholinguistics* (pp. 945–984). San Diego, CA: Academic Press.

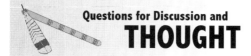

Questions for Discussion and
THOUGHT

1. What actually changes as a language form becomes more automatic?

2. What is a reasonable level of performance to target? Why might you set a goal of 60 to 70 percent instead of 100 percent use?

3. How can we measure progress in the mastery of forms other than grammatical morphemes (e.g., forms that do not have obligatory contexts, such as conjunctions or temporal adverbs)?

4. Imagine two children who both have difficulty with language production but only one of whom has difficulty with sentence comprehension. What can be inferred about the differing nature of their production problems?

Self-Guided Learning
ACTIVITY

Select the child on your caseload that seems to have the greatest number of false starts, self-corrections, pauses, and unfinished utterances. Next time you see this child, tape a short language sample. Take a sheet of paper and write a column of utterance numbers. Now, listen to the tape without transcribing it, and as you listen, count and write down the number of morphemes in each utterance. Listen to the tape one more time and rate each utterance for severity of disruption, on a scale of 1 to 5. For each of the longer utterances, also note whether the utterance is syntactically complex (e.g., 2+ clauses, embedded sentence). Now look at the resulting data. Do the most disrupted utterances tend to be longer? And do they involve sentence complexity?

8 Memory Lessons

I remember as a child being fascinated with books and courses that promised to improve my memory. I suspected they were bogus offers meant only to get my allowance, but I also knew, even then, that memory was a key factor in human function. Moreover, the outcomes seemed promising: less time on homework, fewer lists, more jokes, a bigger vocabulary. As I think about it today, what interests me is that my fascination was with *memory*—not attention, not perception, not reasoning. Those mental processes I took for granted, but not memory. Memory is an aspect of cognition that regularly intrudes into everyday consciousness, and invites theories from all of us.

Given its accessibility and importance, it is surprising that there isn't a longer history of memory studies in the literature on developmental language disorders. Over the last decade, however, researchers have been investigating this area quite energetically.

Working Memory Capacity

Modern views of memory have moved beyond the simple distinction between short-term and long-term storage that was used in my first psychology courses. Models now include *working memory*, a functional space in which data is manipulated as well as stored. One influential theorist, Alan Baddeley (e.g., 1986), divides working memory into three components—*the phonological loop* for temporary storage of auditory material, *the sketchpad* for temporary storage of visual-spatial material, and *the central executive* for control, coordination, and monitoring activities. There is little doubt now that many children with language impairments show capacity limitations in auditory working memory, as evidenced by poor repetition of nonwords, and shorter auditory memory spans on a variety of tasks. Whether these limitations extend to central executive functions is less clear. From a general cognitive viewpoint, there are certainly many tasks for a central executive to carry out in the course of language processing, for example *selecting* the signal to perceive, *calling up* syntactic frames from long-term store, *coordinating* the various knowledge bases required by narratives, *monitoring* one's own comprehension, *testing* hypotheses, and so on. We are just beginning to extend our studies of SLI to these higher-level processes.

53

Thinking About Child Language

Researchers often use a dual-task experiment to look at executive functions. In this type of experiment children are given two simultaneous tasks. They might, for example, be told to categorize and match visual pictures while listening for a buzzer, or remember the position of a cartoon figure while repeating nonsense words. Success on the secondary task is often taken as an indication of how much processing capacity was used up by the primary task. When one task is relatively easy, the child's cognitive systems can perform a second one without difficulty. So, for example, children will be fast to notice the buzzer and press the response button if the visual task is easy. If, however, the first task is difficult, performance on the second task will deteriorate and become worse than it would be if done alone. Other interpretations of dual-task findings stress the coordination of effort that is required, and argue that poor performance reflects inefficient deployment of knowledge, poor monitoring of performance, or difficulties in managing diverse responses. All of these interpretations rest on the assumption that the human mind functions as a limited capacity system. If there is a finite amount of mental energy available at any one moment, a task that requires great concentration or efficiency may use enough of this capacity that little remains for work on a second task. When the traffic is heavy, it's hard to talk and drive.

Working Memory and Language Impairment

Although the line of demarcation between the phonological loop and the central executive is often unclear, activities that go beyond storage to the coordination and manipulation of information are usually attributed to the central executive. Thus, many of the language errors seen in children with specific language impairments (e.g., syntax/morphology tradeoffs or word finding difficulties), point to the possibility of central executive deficits. As part of a larger study on language processing, Ellis Weismer and Thordardottir (2002) explored possible problems with working memory. Their dual task presented children with competing auditory signals: two taped speakers, female in one ear and male in the other, simultaneously gave instructions for moving tokens (e.g., put the white chip on the plate). The children were told to respond first to the woman's instructions, and then to the man's. All of the children found the dual-task condition difficult, and performed quite poorly. Most interesting, however, was the fact that the SLI children were disproportionately affected and showed greater performance decrements than their age peers. This result, while indicating problems in working memory, does not identify their nature. Capacity limits were reached but this could mean either that the children with language impairments had less cognitive energy to distribute, that one or more of the component tasks required a high level of effort, or that the children were less able to coordinate two tasks.

A second study, this one by Lorraine Reggin (2002; Reggin & Johnston, 2003) at the University of British Columbia, takes us closer to being able to choose among these alternatives. She, too, used a dual-task paradigm, but this time one task was visual-spatial and the other was verbal. Twenty-four children age 6 to 9, half with specific language impairments, participated in the study. The auditory-verbal task required children to repeat nonwords of 1 to 4 syllables. The visual-spatial task required them to remember the location of 2 to 6 identical monsters in a 16-cell grid. As is generally true, children in the SLI group had significant difficulty with the longer nonwords. They did not differ from their age peers, however, on the visual task when it was presented singly.

In the dual-task presentation, children had to remember the locations of the monsters over a five-second interval during which they repeated nonwords. All of the children found this combination of memory tasks quite challenging, and performance on the visual task became less accurate. However, unlike Ellis Weismer and Thordardottir (2002), Reggin (2002; Reggin & Johnston, 2003) did *not* find differences between groups. Success in remembering where the monsters had been located declined to the same degree for children with SLI and their age peers.

An important methodological difference between these two studies may explain the different findings. For each of the dual tasks, Reggin only presented items that were at the child's own memory span level, thus equating the difficulty of memory storage across children. No child was asked to remember more than his or her demonstrated capacity. With storage demands controlled, children with SLI seemed able to coordinate performance on the two tasks just as well as the children who did not have language problems. Whatever was needed to monitor memory states and allocate resources so as to maximize recall of the locations seemed to be unimpaired.

Measures of Success...Not Cost

Many functions are attributed to the central executive, and research in this area with children who have SLI has barely begun. As is evident from the two studies summarized here, we can't say for certain whether the central executive is a source of their performance errors or not. Note, however, that whether their problems

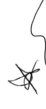

with language processing turn out to be due to reduced storage capabilities, lack of interpretive or generative schemes, or a poorly functioning executive, the end result is the same. Many children with language impairments reach the capacity limits of working memory, particularly auditory working memory, sooner than would be expected for their age, and hence are able to accomplish less mental work than their peers. Do we need to create a course of memory improvement for SLI? And, is it possible?

To answer these intervention questions, think first about the notion of limited capacity. In both of the above studies, children with language impairments were relatively successful in their responses to the first task when it was presented alone. However, the performance decrements that occurred when the second task was added, revealed that this accomplishment had used up much of their available mental energy. Success often hides costs. We can measure success, but it is much more difficult to measure the internal cost of that success. Two children may both succeed on a given task, but one of them may need full concentration and effort to do so while the other child can do the task while watching a soccer game. The true costs may only become visible in a distracting environment, in an inability to move flexibly between tasks, or in a child's failure to complete a hidden, cognitive extension of the more visible primary task. This last point is a crucial one and warrants elaboration. What sort of hidden, secondary tasks might be at jeopardy?

Two of these secondary tasks turn out to be *language learning* and *sense making*. Clearly these tasks are secondary only by virtue of logic and timing, not importance! For a language listener, the primary task is communication, getting the message. If this job exhausts mental capacity, there may be no opportunity to analyze and register the new syntactic pattern or lexeme that the message contained. The opportunity for language learning is lost. The same line of argument applies to sense making, the business of drawing together diverse sorts of information to build a rich, inference-laden, meaning-of-the-whole. Studies of narrative comprehension, for example, have shown that children with SLI have difficulty answering questions about a story when inferences are required. Again, the immediate work of understanding the story facts may consume the available resources and leave children unable to integrate these meanings into a larger whole. Some consequences of capacity limitations are behaviorally evident. We can observe the morphological errors at the end of a complex sentence. But those moments when a new language form is *not* learned or a broader meaning is *not* constructed go largely unnoticed. We only see their cumulative effects in the general language delay.

The research by Ellis Weismer and Thordardottir (2002), Reggin (2002), and others indicates that children with language impairments experience capacity limitations that must impede everyday communication and learning. The research also reminds us of the invisible costs of these memory limitations. There would seem to be ample reason for setting memory improvement as an intervention goal—but how do we go about it? Can we really increase capacity?

Memory Metaphors and Intervention Strategies

Memory improvement, like all interventions, first requires that we understand the nature of the functions we wish to alter. Memory metaphors capture basic elements of this understanding. The most common metaphors evoke images of bins and boxes, refreshed screens, activated circuitry, and railway switchmen. Although these metaphors point to certain relationships and stimulate our thinking about memory processes, none of them leads readily to intervention options. How do we give children bigger bins, increase refreshment rates, increase wattage, or repair switches?

As argued so well by George Miller 40 years ago (1956), the adult working memory span appears to be seven plus or minus two *somethings*. But, these *somethings*, the units of memory, can vary widely in scope and information potential. In the world of language, we might be remembering seven phonetic slices, seven phonemes, seven words, seven phrases, or seven sentences. More importantly, the same acoustic signal can be remembered in any one, or all, of these ways. What is a string of sounds to one person can be a word to someone else—*if* they know the word.

Prior knowledge helps determine *how* we organize events for memory coding. Here, then, is our best opportunity for intervention. The child's mental software (i.e., the scope and automaticity of the knowledge schemes that are used to identify a signal or prepare an action) is a major determinant of working memory capacity, and can be improved in therapy. If we help children learn new, broader-scope patterns, concepts, and routines, they will be better able to manage more information in a given unit of time. By increasing what the child knows about language and how well he or she knows it, we improve the child's capacity for interpreting, learning, and remembering.❖

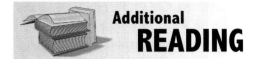

Additional
READING

Baddeley, A. (1986). *Working memory*. Oxford: Oxford University Press.

Miller, G. (1956). The magical number seven, plus or minus two: Some limits on our capacity for processing information. *Psychological Review, 63*, 81–97.

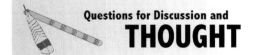

Questions for Discussion and
THOUGHT

1. Does it make sense that you can increase the capacity of the memory "bin" without increasing its size? Can you think of concrete, real-world instances where capacity is not completely determined by size?

2. What determines whether we process speech as successive sounds, words, or sentences?

3. Dual tasks sound exotic until we think of them as just one more instance of *multitasking*. We do it all the time, and with more than two tasks at once. What have you noticed about your own multitasking? What influences success? What strategies, if any, have you developed?

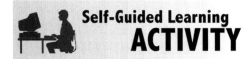

Self-Guided Learning
ACTIVITY

In this essay I argue that we can give children better tools for organizing information, but cannot improve their memory processes directly. What about all those memory improvement courses? Google "memory improvement" and you will find hundreds of search results—books, drugs, nutrition, software, strategies, and yes, courses guaranteed to improve your memory. Spend an hour surfing this motley list. What sorts of strategies are being promoted? Are they usable in therapy with children? Why or why not?

9 Being Smart

A growing body of research on children with specific language impairments (SLI) indicates that they have cognitive processing difficulties as well as language difficulties. Some of the cognitive tasks used in these studies invite the inner use of language, so poor performance could be viewed as the secondary effect of a language disorder. However, performance on other cognitive tasks (e.g., mental rotation or auditory gap detection) is not enhanced by the use of language, and children with SLI have difficulties with these tasks as well.

New Data on Cognitive Processing

A recent study by Nancie Im-Bolter (2003) at York University adds to the evidence on processing limitations. She focused on mental attention and executive processes, the coordinating and organizing actions of the mind that are attributed to working memory. Participants in her study were 90 children, age 7 to 12, half of whom showed language delays of at least 1 SD. The two groups were matched by age, gender, and WISC performance IQ.

Group differences were ultimately found on six of the nine tasks given to each child. Findings from two of the tasks are particularly interesting because they are convincingly nonverbal, and make use of paradigms that seldom, if ever, occur in studies of SLI.

1. **Figural Intersection.** Children were shown a complex pattern of overlaid geometric shapes, and alongside them, a set of the single shapes that made up the pattern. The task was to indicate the point in the pattern at which all of the individual shapes intersected. Children in the SLI group were less accurate than their age peers.

2. **Antisaccade.** Children stared at a fixation point (plus sign) in the middle of the computer screen for a second or two. Then a small square appeared briefly (225 milliseconds) on one side of the screen or the other. The screen went blank for 50 milliseconds and then an arrow appeared on the opposite side of the screen for 100 milliseconds. The children were asked to indicate which direction the arrow had pointed. The challenge in this task is to inhibit the natural desire to look at the square and to stay focused on the fixation point. If you look at the square instead of leaving it in

peripheral vision, there is not enough time to refocus on the arrow before it disappears. Ample training trials were provided. Children with SLI were again less accurate in their judgments about the direction of the arrow, 60 percent versus 72 percent. Their performance was strong enough to show that they understood the task, but they seemed to have difficulty in attending to the fixation point.

From a real-world point of view, these tasks are pretty artificial. However, they do seem to require the same sorts of mental activity that we need for everyday problem solving, that is, attentive and planful processing of perceptual information. So here in the Im-Bolton (2003) data, we find further evidence that children with specific language impairments have cognitive processing difficulties that are neither specific nor exclusively linguistic.

A Puzzle

The enigma I have lived with for over a decade is this: if children with SLI do have pervasive general cognitive processing problems, how can they be smart? It has seemed to me, and to others who have criticized my cognitivist position, that general cognitive processing problems, if present, should affect all intellectual functions and preclude being smart. Yet, clinical experience tells us that this is just what SLI children are—smart! How do we reconcile the two data sets of the experimental research and the clinical observation? To be sure, some SLI children "fade" as they continue into the later school years. Their normal range nonverbal IQ scores begin to decline as the intellectual tasks expected for their age depend more and more on verbal skills or experience. However, not all children with SLI show this decline.

New Data on Numerical Reasoning

Confirmation that indeed some children with SLI are able to handle age-appropriate reasoning tasks comes from Great Britain. Over the last few years, Chris Donlan at University College has conducted a project entitled "Number Talk," looking at number knowledge and numerical reasoning in 60 eight-year-olds with SLI (2003). Each of these children was matched with a younger child (age 6) by language level, as well as with an age peer. All 180 participants earned normal range nonverbal IQ on the Ravens Progressive Matrices.

The Number Talk battery included tests of many lower-level mathematical skills—counting; writing numerals from dictation; giving sums for single digit addition such as 2 + 3; and pointing to pictures of quantities that were more, most, fewer, etc. On all of these tasks, the children with SLI performed much like their language peers and significantly less well than their age peers. The one higher-level task was an exception to this rule. The task assessed the child's understanding of commutativity, the principle that if A + B = V, then B + A = V. Children were asked to help a Martian teacher mark some papers. The teacher had marked one of a pair of equations as being correct and the child had to decide if the second equation was also correct. On this conceptual task, the children with SLI outperformed their language peers and actually scored in the range of their age peers. Barb Fazio found similar conceptual strengths in her studies of numerical reasoning; her work is described in Essay 26.

This body of data, in contrast to the data from the visual perceptual tasks, tells us that in spite of their processing difficulties, children with specific language impairments can indeed be smart. How can we reconcile these two views, which are both empirically grounded?

Operational Intelligence Revisited

I began to see some light on this issue in a long conversation with Donlan's research associate, Elizabeth Newton. Prior to working on Number Talk, she had conducted research on higher-level reasoning processes in adults. During a presentation to my lab group, Newton gave us one of the classic reasoning tasks. She showed us four cards, each with a single number on one side and a single letter on the other. Initially we saw only one side of each card: R, H, 4, 7. Then, she posed her question. "Which card(s) would you need to turn over to find out if this set conforms to the rule: All cards with R have a 4 on the other side?" The R card was the simple first choice, but when Liz told us to choose another card from the set, things got more interesting. Some of us were initially drawn to the 4 instead of the correct card, the 7. (Think about it, then read the note at the end of the essay.) As Liz discussed the logic of this problem, I realized that's what had been missing in my picture of SLI—logic!

Complex reasoning tasks involve at least five types of mental activity:

• Formulation of a plan

• Perception of the facts

- Internal representation of these facts

- Coordination and allocation of resources

- Logical and spatial/temporal/causal operations

Researchers in the area of language disorders are typically referring to the middle three types of activity when they talk about cognitive processing and, indeed, children with SLI seem to have difficulties with each of them. But perception, real-time representation, and resource allocation are not the whole story—there are still the *plan* and the *operations*. Little if any research on language disorders has addressed these aspects of cognition, but they may be the keys to being smart.

I know virtually nothing about the development of planfulness and related areas of metacognition, so I have added this topic to my list of learning goals. Logic, on the other hand, is an old friend. For more than five years of my doctoral program, I attended a weekly seminar on the theories of the Swiss psychologist Jean Piaget. As we studied his work, I had many opportunities to reflect on the nature of higher level reasoning processes. At the heart of Piaget's theory is the idea that intelligent thought consists of internalized mental actions such as combining, dissociating, ordering, and transforming. These operations are learned singly, and with particular material experiences, but eventually they become systematized and content free.

By the school years, children know that dogs and cats *combine* into the superordinate class of animals. They also know they can *remove* the cats from the animals and have a coherent subclass. By the school years, children also know that they can transform a ball of clay into a pancake, and that they can transform the clay pancake into a ball. Piaget argued that these superficially different bodies of knowledge are logically similar in that they both involve reversibility. If $A + B = X$, then $X - B = A$. Likewise, if $A \rightarrow B$, then $B \rightarrow A$. His point wasn't merely that mental actions could be undone, but that each mental operation actually implied an entire set of potential operations that made up a system of mental actions to be considered simultaneously. These mental systems serve as the basis for predicting outcomes and analyzing relationships and are the essence of intelligent reasoning.

Being Smart

If children with SLI were able to construct these abstract systems of mental operations at a normal or near normal age, they would have the tools needed for diverse reasoning tasks. They would also have a way to be smart. Their challenge is to *plan, perceive, represent,* and *allocate* in such a fashion that they still have the resources needed for operational thinking. As clinicians and teachers, that is our challenge as well. What can we do to minimize the cost of processing so that the children with SLI have a chance to be smart? Two cognitive principles will help us reach that goal.

1. **Perception is a two-way process.** Our perception of any event depends on the sensory information we receive *and* on our predictions about what the nature of that information should be. Psychologists sometimes refer to these aspects of perception as *bottom-up* and *top-down* processes. We are used to thinking about the acoustic signal aspects of speech production, or the visual scanning needed for fluent reading, but we sometimes forget that our knowledge of speech sounds, letter shapes, words, and sentence patterns also influences our perception. In a noisy room, for example, we can fill in the bits of signal that we don't actually hear because we know what should be there.

   The two-way nature of perceptual processes gives us two ways to intervene. We can help children focus on the important auditory or visual data either by making the data more salient (e.g., louder or bolder) or by preparing children ahead of time with the words and ideas they will need to guide perception. For example, speech perception in the classroom can be improved either by moving children with SLI to the front of the room, or by teaching them the vocabulary they will need for the next social studies unit. These may not be new ideas, but the important point here is that whenever we can simplify the perceptual task, we also increase the resources available for other mental work.

2. **Familiar mental schemes are less costly to use.** As schemes are repeatedly used, they become familiar, automatic, and efficient to use. But before a conceptual or reasoning scheme can become familiar, it must be learned in the first place. We can speed children on this learning path by introducing new concepts and operations in the most accessible manner with visual and manipulable learning aids. In Fazio's (1994) study of numerical reasoning, for example, she encouraged the children with SLI to use their fingers to aid in calculations. In Kamhi's (1981) study of operational intelligence, the

children did well on a spatial ordering task in which they could actually move the materials around.

Particularly dramatic evidence of the efficacy of visual and manipulable cues is seen in the Kamhi et al. (1990) study of analogical reasoning. Children with SLI were presented with the classical reasoning task about the farmer, the fox, the goose, the corn, and the boat. The boat is too small for the farmer to transport more than one item at a time across the river. The challenge is to keep the goose away from the corn and the fox away from the goose and still get everyone across the river. Half of the children were taught with visual props that they could move around on the table, as well as with verbal explanations. These children learned the abstract structure of the solution to this task three times faster than the children who only heard the verbal explanations. Children in the visual-props condition were then able to apply the same logic to an entirely different puzzle, one that involved moving rings on and off of pegs. In the real world, learning the basic reasoning schemes in an efficient and rapid manner will leave children with more time for exploration and practice, making it more likely that the new concepts and operations will become familiar tools for thought.

For over a decade, I have been thinking about ways to help children with language impairments compensate for processing limitations, but I had not really considered the relationships between processing deficits and complex reasoning. The hypothesis that I've presented here is that children with SLI can be smart because they are able to construct and use abstract operations of the Piagetian sort. They are frequently impeded in their use of these logical and infralogical schemes, however, by the costs of perception, representation, and resource coordination. If we can increase their effectiveness in these early phases of reasoning, they will be able to use whatever operations they have available to solve the problem. This hypothesis obviously needs further research support and elaboration. But even now it may be useful as you teach children with SLI and try to explain their learning needs to families and educators.❖

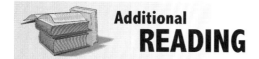

Additional
READING

Gardner, H. (1993). *Frames of mind: The theory of multiple intelligences* (10th ed.). New York: Basic Books.

Hamilton, C., Coates, R., & Heffernan, T. (2003). What develops in visuo-spatial working memory development? *European Journal of Cognitive Psychology, 15*(1), 43–69.

Mayer, R., & Anderson, R. (1991). Animations need narrations: An experimental test of a dual-coding hypothesis. *Journal of Educational Psychology, 83*(4), 484–490.

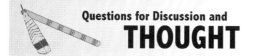

Questions for Discussion and
THOUGHT

1. According to Howard Gardner, we have not one intelligence, but many different ways of perceiving and understanding the world. His initial list includes verbal, logical, spatial, interpersonal, intrapersonal, musical, and kinesthetic intelligences. In his view, an individual's abilities may differ markedly from area to area, and there are many different ways to be smart. Is Gardner's view incompatible with the ideas in this essay? Can they be reconciled?

2. In this essay I suggest ways to improve perception and streamline the acquisition of new interpretive schemes. What about maintaining the facts once they are perceived? Brainstorm some ways to help children keep the facts in mind so that they can reason about them.

3. Arithmetic problems that are presented verbally are particularly difficult for children with language impairments. Find a Grade 5 or Grade 6 math book and turn to a section that has a set of these word problems. Brainstorm some ways to use props to help children solve them. Write down the various ideas as they emerge. Then, reflect on these teaching strategies. What sort of support are you providing? Memory aids? Visualization of a sequence of operations? Or what?

Self-Guided Learning
ACTIVITIES

1. **Try with preschool children.** Find a description of Piaget's basic conservation tasks of matter and number, and administer them to several four-year-olds on your caseload (older fours would be best). Try to predict ahead of time which children will do better, based on your past observations of their reasoning and language abilities. Were you right? Try changing the materials (e.g., poker chips versus toy cars). Does performance change?

   See The PsiCafe (www.psy.pdx.edu/PsiCafe) for a description of the tasks. From the *Inside the PsiCafe* menu bar, click *Key Theorists and Theories,* then click to browse per *The theorists' LAST name,* click *Piaget, Jean.* From the right-hand column LINKS TO, click *Overheads/Images,* then select *Piaget's Conservation Tasks.*

2. **Try with school-age children.** The guessing game Twenty Questions requires logical reasoning, mostly about class inclusion relations. It also requires holding many facts in mind. Prepare a version of the game with a restricted set of targets and some sort of external memory aids. Try teaching a child with SLI (MA 9+) how to play this game.

NOTE: Regarding the logic problem: The rule says "All cards with R have a 4 on the other side." The reverse is not necessarily true. There may be cards with a 4 that do not have an R. All we are interested in is whether cards that do have an R also have a 4. The only possible exception to the rule in this set of cards would be the 7. If it has an R on the other side, the set would not fit the rule; if it does not have an R on the other side, the set does fit the rule.

10 Never a Poet

I remember clearly the day I found myself saying to a mother, "Brian will never be a poet, but he definitely will learn to talk." I was trying to convey the complicated two-pronged prognosis for preschool language impairment: first, that most children will learn to express themselves with words; and second, that they are likely to have continuing weakness in language abilities. This is often difficult for parents and teachers to understand, since they focus so completely on speech itself, and treat the lack of speech as the problem rather than as a symptom. From their vantage point, children who talk have been cured.

The fate of the five-year-olds just entering kindergarten illustrates the potential cost of this misunderstanding. Take the case of Andy. He has been in kindergarten for four weeks and the school team just met to discuss his educational programming. Despite the fact that tests by his preschool SLP indicated a two-year expressive and receptive language delay, his teacher reports that Andy is now doing well. He sits in groups with the other children and takes his turn at circle time. She understands his speech and is confident he understands the classroom discourse. However, last year two similarly impaired children who were also "doing well" with this teacher in the fall, experienced total classroom failure in the spring, and spent increasing periods of the day in the "time out" room. Does this teacher have poor judgment, or is something else going on? How likely is it that Andy's language problem has resolved? Should the SLP be concerned?

Late Talkers

Over the last decade, two lines of research have investigated the outcomes of early language impairment. One group of studies has looked at Late Talkers (Paul, 1991), the other at children with specific language impairments. At first these two bodies of research seem to be telling rather different stories, but I believe the differences are more apparent than real. Let's collect a few facts.

Late Talkers were originally defined as children between the ages of 18 and 24 months who lacked age-appropriate verbal skills. By the current diagnostic rule of thumb, a child at 2;0 should either have a 50-word productive vocabulary or be combining words, or both. Late Talkers fail to meet this criterion despite relatively normal cognitive and social development. Groups of such children have now been followed for more than five years in Portland, Madison, Pennsylvania, San Diego, and New York. The different projects have had somewhat different agendas, but these two important findings are reported by virtually all of them:

- 45 to 60 percent of toddlers identified as Late Talkers outgrow their language delays by age 4.

- The children with continuing problems are very likely to have shown early delays in language *comprehension* as well as expression.

As children in these longitudinal studies have grown older, those with persistent problems exactly fit the criteria for specific language impairment. This has caused some confusion in the popular press with writers treating the "recovery" rates seen for Late Talkers (by definition, diagnosed at age 2), as if they applied to all preschoolers with language delays including those identified as having SLI at ages 3 or 4. This is definitely not the case, as we will see next in a set of studies from Great Britain.

Longitudinal Studies of Specific Language Impairment

The work of Bishop and Edmundson (1987) is often cited as proof that many preschoolers with language impairment do recover. This research team tested 64 children with language impairments and normal nonverbal IQ on three occasions over an 18-month period. They used a battery of standardized tests that assessed phonological, vocabulary, and grammatical knowledge as well as verbal reasoning abilities. Before summarizing the findings, several methodological features of this study deserve mention. First, the researchers did not use test results to decide whether a child fit into their study, but instead used SLP referrals. A small number of their participants turned out to be not actually impaired. They also decided to include children who had phonological problems, but no other difficulties with language. While phonology is certainly a part of language, such children are not commonly included in samples of SLI. The findings I will summarize here focus on the 55 children that remain when these two groups are excluded.

Bishop and Edmundson's goal was to determine the percentage of children who had language impairments at age 4 but satisfactory language at age 5;6. To be judged "satisfactory," a child could not score below the 10th percentile in more than one language domain. When all the testing was over, the researchers concluded that 35 percent of the children who had been diagnosed as having a specific language impairment at age 4 had satisfactory language by age 5;6. This figure is of course higher (41 percent) if we throw the phonologically impaired children back into the mix. The researchers argue further that recovery was most likely to be seen in children who had mild semantic/comprehension problems. But ceiling effects on the pertinent tests call this conclusion into question. While somewhat lower than the recovery rate reported for Late Talkers, the Bishop and Edmundson figure was still encouraging: at age 4, one in three preschoolers with normal nonverbal intelligence and language delays could be expected to catch up.

Bishop and her colleagues recently published a follow-up to the original study (Stothard et al., 1998). Forty-nine children who had been part of the first project were again given a battery of language and cognitive tests, this time at age 15. The new findings are sobering. Only 13 percent of the children who had impaired language at both age 4 and 5;6 had satisfactory language at age 15. Moreover, 93 percent of them were at least three years behind in reading achievement. An equally dramatic finding was that 32 percent of the children who had been judged to have a resolved SLI at age 5;6 were again showing impaired language at age 15, and 52 percent of them were more than three years behind in reading achievement. For these children, recovery at age 5;6 had turned out to be ephemeral.

This picture of continuing impairment is well in line with longitudinal studies in Canada (Young et al., 2002) and the United States (Tomblin et al., 1992). The message in these studies is clear. Children who have difficulty learning their first language have a serious and persistent disability. The human mind has evolved to learn to talk, so we shouldn't be surprised to find that failure to learn language is not a trivial problem. But what about the teacher and Andy, and for that matter, the earlier Bishop and Edmundson (1987) findings? What happens to make us believe that the five-year-olds with histories of language impairment have been cured?

Illusory Recovery from Language Impairment

Scarborough and Dobrich (1990) may have solved the puzzle of the children "cured at five." Based on their longitudinal data from a study of dyslexia, they argue that there is a plateau in the normal course of language learning that occurs around 45 to 60 months of age, at least as measured by traditional tools (solid line in graph). Children with SLI (dotted line) can catch up with their age peers during this period, but this recovery is illusory. Shortly after the two curves make contact, the normally developing children begin to forge ahead on new language learning challenges, and the children with SLI remain in the plateau zone, once again left

Thinking About Child Language

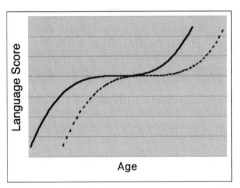

Language Score

Age

behind. It is a bit of bad luck for Andy and the many SLPs who serve preschoolers that the point at which the two developmental curves temporarily join is in kindergarten. Andy's teacher may be right. He may be doing fine. But the research cited above, along with the notion of illusory recovery, suggests that we should be quite cautious in predicting long-term success. It may be that by providing language intervention during the early kindergarten period, even when children seem to have caught up with their peers, we can avoid later classroom failure. Federal funding policies in the United States now provide for such "early intervening" without assignment to a traditional diagnostic category (Boswell, 2005). Other countries may follow suit. At the least, close observation and a language assessment midyear will help us make better educational decisions for children with histories of preschool language impairment.

Fast Facts

As SLPs and educators, we increasingly find ourselves having to advocate for language intervention services. The next time you talk with political and educational policymakers, the following figures derived from the Stothard et al. (1998) data may prove useful. (Note that the figures based on this Great Britain study are approximate, since they attempt to exclude children who only showed phonological difficulties.)

- Two out of three 4-year-olds with specific language disorder will continue to have oral language difficulties at age 15.

- Three out of four 4-year-olds with specific language disorder will be three or more years behind in reading at age 15.

As is clear from these numbers, we can't promise cures, but we can promise that the children we work with will learn language sooner and faster than they would without our support. They may not reach the levels of achievement seen in their peers, and they may never be poets. They will, however, learn language, and the new language they bring to the classroom will enable further learning.❖

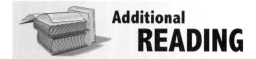

Additional
READING

Tomblin, J. B., Freese, P., & Records, N. (1992). Diagnosing specific language impairment in adults for the purposes of pedigree analysis. *Journal of Speech and Hearing Research, 35,* 832–843.

Young, A., Beitchman, J., Johnson, C., Douglas, L., Atkinson, L., Escobar, M., et al. (2002). Young adult academic outcomes in a longitudinal sample of early identified language impaired and control children. *Journal of Child Psychology and Psychiatry and Allied Disciplines, 43,* 635–646.

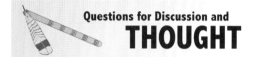

Questions for Discussion and
THOUGHT

1. Although it would explain our difficulties in program decisions for five-year-olds, the notion of a plateau in language learning is counterintuitive. Children certainly show growth spurts in various domains, but they seldom totally stop making progress. In what way(s) could language be developing in the kindergarten years without these changes showing up in test scores?

2. What sort of data might convince a skeptical teacher that a child does indeed have a language problem?

3. Why does the prognosis for a child with significant language delay depend on the child's age at diagnosis? Discuss the likelihood and sufficiency of the following explanations: differences in severity, treatment effects, or misdiagnosis.

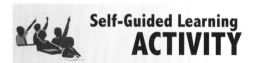

Self-Guided Learning
ACTIVITY

For school SLPs. Keep a record of the next three children in kindergarten or grade 1 with a history of speech-language services that you decide not to treat. At the end of 6 months and 12 months, observe the child in the classroom, talk to the teacher, and administer a test or two. Do the children indeed seem to have recovered?

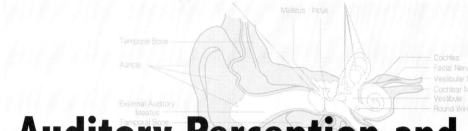

Auditory Perception and Language Disorder

Human language is most commonly learned from speech and therefore involves audition. Logically, of course, this does not mean that language learning disorders are necessarily the result of auditory deficits, but that is certainly a good possibility. There is now a large body of research on auditory perceptual deficits in children with SLI, and I have concluded that at least one subgroup of these children does have difficulty with nonverbal auditory perceptual tasks. I am even comfortable with the idea that this difficulty has something to do with poor language learning. I am not convinced, however, that the source of either the perceptual or the language problem is actually auditory.

As you read the essays in this section, you will have the chance to think about auditory explanations for impaired language learning. The section begins with an essay about language comprehension, and reminds us of the top-down as well as bottom-up nature of this process. Then, I offer my latest thoughts on central auditory processing disorder (a perpetual item on the ASHA agenda), and share some wise self-diagnoses from a 10-year-old. Along the way, we'll find several reasons to wonder whether audition is the key to language learning disorders at all.

11 More Than a Crash-Test Dummy

While describing her research on speech perception in a colloquium at our university, a visiting audiologist/psychoacoustician repeatedly referred to the use of KEMAR. When we ignorant SLPs asked what this meant, we learned that KEMAR is the audiologists' version of a crash-test dummy. "He" is a synthetic head and torso complete with ear canals and pinnae, used to collect and relay multisource acoustic signals. Researchers who utilize KEMAR do so because he can't walk and doesn't turn his head, making it possible to control those aspects of the signal that depend on position and orientation. Unfortunately, KEMAR also has no brain, which seems to me to be a major drawback when studying human perception. The old view of a one-way flow of data from ear to brain has, after all, been replaced by a more interactive one in which knowledge and expectation inevitably participate in perceptual experience.

We may not use dummy listeners, but sometimes we treat our clients as if they, too, had a pair of pinnae and ear canals and nothing in between. We talk about the auditory problems of children with language impairments as if audition were simply a peripheral, sensory process. And we talk about comprehension problems as if they were primarily auditory, forgetting about the role of language knowledge, selective attention, or the efforts of the listener to make meaning. Recent studies of language comprehension invite us to think about this aspect of language use in a more complex way.

The Many Faces of Language Comprehension

Before looking at the studies, it might be useful to reflect a moment on what we mean when we talk about comprehension. Clinicians seem to use the phrase *language comprehension* to refer to a number of different mental tasks and states. I've had SLPs say to me that they always begin with comprehension activities when addressing a new language target. Further questioning reveals, however, that all they mean to be saying is that the child is not required to talk. Since we don't know whether or not the child is actually focused on getting the message, it would be more accurate to call these *not-talking* activities or *exposure* activities, rather than comprehension activities.

75

Thinking About Child Language

At other times, SLPs have told me that children learn new forms through comprehension. Again, this is only partially true. While language-learning events indeed must begin with estimates of meaning, this by itself is not enough. In order to learn something new, children must also analyze the language forms that they have just heard so that they can store the relationships between forms and meanings. At still other times, I've heard SLPs discuss children who don't yet know some language form, but nevertheless comprehend it. As we talk further, it turns out that they have in mind some nonverbal representation of a concept or fact.

In these examples the same word is being used to refer to four vastly different mental events: listening, figuring out what someone means, analyzing new language forms, and having knowledge of a concept. Since the legitimate domain of comprehension is already complex, referring to all of these mental tasks and states as instances of comprehension seems only to confuse matters.

There are three mental tasks that I think deserve to be called comprehension. First, there is the process of figuring out the message that is being directly expressed in words. Second, there is the process of determining a larger message of the whole, of putting all the sentential pieces together to get the bigger picture, a process that is sometimes called *constructive comprehension*. And finally, there is comprehension monitoring, the ongoing evaluation of one's own success in getting the message. Each of these mental tasks has its own internal complexity, but we can learn much even at this rather general level of description.

Constructive Comprehension

Researchers in Great Britain have conducted two studies that have bearing on our understanding of constructive comprehension, studies that were motivated in large part by an interest in children with semantic-pragmatic disorders. The goal of the studies was to determine whether the inappropriate patterns of language use seen in these children stemmed from an inability to understand language in an integrated fashion. Letts and Leinonen's (2001) study focused on inferential meaning. In their experimental tasks, children were asked to look at a series of pictures and answer seven questions of the following types:

- Two questions concerned matters of fact (e.g., What is the woman doing?)

- Three questions required an inferential judgment based on evidence in the picture (e.g., Are these three friends?)

- One question asked the child to infer a person's feelings (e.g. How does he feel?)

- One question invited problem solving (e.g., What do you think the lady should do?)

For each of the inferential questions, the researchers also asked the child to provide a reason for the inference.

Note that this task attempts to get at some of the basic reasoning skills that underlie constructive comprehension. The use of pictures rather than verbal texts enabled children to access the events without decoding symbols, and to work with information that did not disappear into silence. The researchers also used the same simple syntactic forms in the inferential questions as were in the descriptive questions. Together, these features reduced (but did not totally remove) the constraints of language ability and memory, and provided a more direct look at inferencing skills.

Three age groups participated in this study: a group of 7- to 10-year-olds with language impairment, half of whom also showed pragmatic deficits; a group of normally developing 6- to 8-year-olds; and a group of normally developing 16- to 17-year-olds.

Virtually everyone answered all of the descriptive questions correctly. The older teens were more likely than other participants to talk about the strength of the evidence and to argue that a simple *yes/no* answer to the inferential questions was not possible. There were no further group differences on inferencing. Where the groups did differ was in explaining their inferences. The language-impaired children gave twice as many inadequate explanations as the other groups, either saying nothing at all, saying merely, "because," or giving an answer that was irrelevant or unintelligible. Interestingly, there were no differences within the impaired group; the presence or absence of pragmatic problems did not, in fact, predict performance on the inference task.

The second study looked at inferences drawn after listening to oral stories. Norbury and Bishop (2002) asked children to answer questions about each of five stories. There were three types of questions:

- Questions about information that had been directly provided

- Questions that required text connecting inferences drawn from adjacent sentences

- Questions that required gap-filling inferences in which the child's own knowledge needed to be integrated with information in the text

In addition to the story task, participants also completed a digit-span task, a receptive language test (either vocabulary or grammar), and a sentence imitation task. All of the participating children were around age 9, but could be divided by diagnosis into four groups: specific language impairment (SLI), autism, pragmatic impairment (PI), or normally developing (ND).

At first pass, the results of the story-comprehension task were surprising. All of the children found the gap-filling inferences the most difficult, but there was little difference in the group means. In a secondary analysis, the researchers identified those individual children who had low story-comprehension scores. Twenty-five percent of the SLI group, 33 percent of the PI group, and 50 percent of the autism group fell below the lowest ND score. But when the information from the receptive language tests was factored in, these group differences disappeared. The troubles with story comprehension seemed to reflect gaps in vocabulary and syntax knowledge rather than difficulties with drawing inference.

Despite the initial lack of group differences, Norbury and Bishop (2002) tried one further analysis. They invented an inference deficit score that indicated whether a child's answers to the inference questions were better or worse than answers to questions for which the information had been given directly. This analysis was different than the preceding one because it used within-child comparisons and looked at inferencing in a relative fashion. It didn't matter whether the child's language level was severely delayed or mildly delayed, or whether the child made many comprehension errors or just a few. All that mattered was the relative difficulty of inferencing, that is, whether or not the questions that required inferences were more difficult than those that did not. This analysis did reveal a relationship between diagnostic group and story comprehension: more children (70 percent) in the autistic group had particular difficulties with inference than was true for children in the other clinical groups (17 to 25 percent). The researchers emphasize, however, that there were some children in each group who showed no special problem with inference. Interestingly, comparisons of children who did and did not show an inference deficit indicated no difference in memory, language, or performance IQ test scores.

The Bottom Line

So where does this leave us? I see three important conclusions that can be drawn from these two studies. First, it is clear from the Norbury and Bishop (2002) analysis that there are indeed some children who have special difficulty in constructing the big picture meanings from an oral text. These children may understand all of the information that is directly given, but their ability to draw inferential meanings is limited. However—and this is the second point—both studies indicate that our diagnostic categories do not do an adequate job of identifying these children. Any clinical decisions about which children have difficulty with this aspect of language comprehension can only be made on a child-by-child basis. It is worth noting here that many of the earlier reports of group deficits in inferencing have been based on comparisons of group means and have not paid attention to the heterogeneity within groups.

Finally—and the conclusion I find most interesting—these studies indicate that inferencing problems, when they exist, are not tied to nonverbal IQ, severity of language delay (test scores), or simple auditory memory span. In fact, the Letts and Leinonen (2001) results suggest that the problems some children have in constructing the larger meanings implicit in an oral text may not be due to problems with inferencing at all, since the children in that study were quite successful with inferences that were based on pictures rather than text.

So what is left? We obviously need further research before we will understand the difficulties that some children have with inference, but one suggestion made by both of these research teams is intriguing: that deficits in inferencing are a consequence of higher-level limitations in working memory and/or language processing. In order to draw inferences by reading between the lines, or integrate stored knowledge with the information in a text, the listener must keep several propositions in mind at once, then analyze and evaluate potential relationships between them. Capacity limitations in verbal working memory would certainly make this task more difficult.

Intervention Ideas

Whatever their origin may be, difficulties with inference can cause classroom challenges and compromise a child's ability to use language for learning. Although there are as yet no intervention studies focused on inferences from oral text, there has been at least one intervention study looking at inferences from printed text.

Yuill and Oakhill (1988) report dramatic improvements in reading comprehension scores following only seven sessions of direct instruction on text inferencing. Oral text may present greater challenges, especially for children with cognitive processing limitations, but this study is nevertheless encouraging.

I am indebted to my former student Wanda Yee for her analysis of treatment options. Working from within a limited capacity model of language processing, she concluded that there are three strategies SLPs can use to help children improve their constructive text comprehension.

1. We can reduce the memory requirements of the text itself either by decreasing language complexity or by providing language practice so that comprehension processes become more automatic and require fewer mental resources. This would free up the memory and attentional resources needed for the comparisons and analysis inherent in inferencing.

2. We can increase children's text processing resources by helping them acquire new language knowledge. With a broader array of parsing and interpretive options, children will again spend less resources figuring out the basic meaning of the text and have more resources for constructing the gist of the whole.

3. We can encourage and guide constructive comprehension by direct instruction, asking questions about a text, making predictions from a text, visually mapping text meanings, and making inferences of all types.

Back to the Crash-Test Dummy

I opened this essay with some thoughts about the nature of research on speech perception and language comprehension. Sometimes it seems like the world of language is just too complicated and uncertain. The studies of inference certainly raised many questions, and at times like these, we may wish that all we had to worry about was KEMAR—no brain, just ears and a head. It's worth remembering at such times that what we study is ultimately ourselves. It may be good to study a KEMAR…but no one wants to be one. We revel daily in the richness of language, and we work to give our kids that same experience.❖

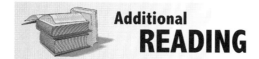

Additional
READING

Gillam, R. B. (1996). Putting memory to work in language intervention: Implications for practitioners. *Topics in Language Disorders, 18,* 72–79.

Johnston, J., & Welsh, E. (2000). Comprehension of "because" and "so": The role of prior event representation. *First Language, 20,* 291–304.

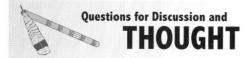

Questions for Discussion and
THOUGHT

1. What is a limited capacity system? Can you think of any evidence that supports the view that language processing takes place in such a system? What would be the opposing point(s) of view?

2. This essay mentions four different mental activities that all have been called *comprehension* by SLPs. Talk further about these four activities, thinking particularly about the goals and knowledge requirements for each one.

3. Imagine a school-age child who has difficulty in drawing inferences from spoken texts (e.g., oral stories, classroom lectures, or explanations). How do you think that a parent or a teacher would describe such a child? What could they say that would alert you to the likelihood that the child has difficulty with inferencing?

4. Is language comprehension easier than language formulation? Does age, language level, or the nature of the message influence your answer to this question? How?

Self-Guided Learning
ACTIVITIES

1. **Try with preschool children.** Although children with mental ages in the 3 to 5 year range may have difficulty drawing inferences from text, they can take a step in that direction by going beyond the facts of the story in other ways. For example, they can make predictions about what will happen next, or imagine what a character looks like or is feeling. Use the exercise that is suggested for school-age children, but change the inference questions into more open-ended questions of this type.

2. **Try with school-age children.** Select three stories differing in length and complexity from a published source such as The Listening Test (a test of text comprehension) or the Test of Narrative Language (longer texts). Write four questions for each story, two dealing with facts and two requiring inference. Read the stories to children on your caseload who have low scores on tests of vocabulary comprehension or sentence comprehension. If a child makes any comprehension errors, are they more likely to occur on inference items or on fact items?

12 CAPD: 20 Years of Debate and Still Counting

In 1995 the American Speech-Language-Hearing Association (ASHA) held an interdisciplinary conference on central auditory processing disorder (CAPD or APD) and asked experts across North America to contribute state-of-the-art research papers. I was one of a group of audiologists, hearing scientists, psychologists, and speech-language pathologists who, following the conference, were locked in a hotel room and asked to produce a consensus paper. Despite wide differences in perspective, we did find substantial areas of agreement. The resultant paper was published as an ASHA technical report (Catts et al., 1996) but was never adopted as official policy.

I'll return to the content of that report in a moment, but its historical context is equally interesting. The 1995 effort was actually the fourth or fifth in a series of ASHA working groups on CAPD extending back into the early 1980s. In 2004 there was yet another. This time, following two years of discussion, a group of audiologists posted a new CAPD position paper for review by ASHA members. It offered no new science, but presented a radically different view of CAPD than the one constructed by our consensus group. The 2004 paper was subsequently approved as an official ASHA policy statement by the Audiology/Hearing Science Assembly (ASHA, 2005a). What is going on here? What is the nature of the debates surrounding CAPD? And why do they continue to boil?

The Audiological View

My search for answers to these questions led me first to various sources available or listed on the Web. Here are some of the definitions that I found:

- Auditory processing is a term used to describe what happens when your brain recognizes and interprets the sounds around you…The disorder part of auditory processing disorder means that something is adversely affecting the processing or interpretation of the information…The cause of APD is often unknown. In children, [it] may be associated with conditions such as dyslexia, attention-deficit/hyperactivity disorder, autism, specific language impairment, or developmental delay. (National Institutes of Health, 2004).

- CAPD results from dysfunction of processes dedicated to audition; however, CAPD also may coexist with a more global dysfunction that affects performance across modalities, such as attention deficit, neural timing deficit, or language representation deficit (Chermak et al., 1999).

- Many neurocognitive functions are involved in the processing of auditory information. Some are specific to the processing of acoustic signals, while others are more global…(e.g., attention, memory, language representation). However, these latter functions are considered components of auditory processing when they are involved in the processing of auditory information (Schminky & Baran, 2000 p. 41).

- Central auditory processing disorder occurs when the ear and the brain do not coordinate fully…[There are] five main problem areas that can affect both home and school activities in children with CAPD.

1. Auditory Figure-Ground Problems [e.g.] "when the child cannot pay attention when there is noise in the background."

2. Auditory Memory Problems [e.g.] "when the child has difficulty remembering information such as directions."

3. Auditory Discrimination Problems [e.g.] "when the child has difficulty hearing the difference between sounds or words that are similar."

4. Auditory Attention Problems [e.g.] "when the child cannot maintain focus for listening."

5. Auditory Cohesion Problems [e.g.] "drawing inferences from conversations, understanding riddles or comprehending verbal math problems — require heightened auditory processing and language levels" (Kidshealth, 2004).

These excerpts convey the themes that distinguish what I will call the audiological view of CAPD. Experts working within this perspective believe that: (1) the mental events involved in the processing of acoustic information are *best* viewed as auditory, (2) CAPD may coexist with other conditions but is *importantly* distinct from them, and (3) the academic, language, and attentional problems seen in many children are actually a manifestation, or result of, CAPD.

I know of no one who disputes the existence of central auditory processing disorders or doubts that, when present, they significantly affect learning and communication. The causal equation cannot, however, be reversed. Difficulty with communication, attention, or learning tasks does not necessarily point to CAPD, even when there is an auditory signal. Moreover, in the case of children, it has proven difficult to demonstrate the uniquely auditory nature of the condition. In fact, the new ASHA policy (ASHA, 2005a) concludes that "any definition of APD that would require complete modality-specificity as a diagnostic criterion is neurophysiologically untenable," and that "one-to-one correspondence between deficits in fundamental, discrete auditory processes and language, learning, and related sequelae may be difficult to demonstrate across large groups of diverse subjects." The working group nevertheless goes on to argue that APD is "best viewed as a deficit in neural processing of auditory stimuli that may coexist with, but is not the result of, dysfunction in other modalities."

The Language View

The traditional opposition in the CAPD debate has been the "language" camp, peopled mostly by speech-language pathologists. For them, the learning and communication problems seen in many school-age children are a source, rather than a consequence, of auditory difficulties.

A research study in Munich (Uwer et al., 2002) speaks to this possibility. Forty-two children with specific language impairment, age 5 to 10, were tested for auditory functions with two sorts of stimuli: tones and CV syllables. Testing was conducted with both passive and active auditory perceptual tasks: electrophysiological procedures (mismatched negativity, MMN) and discriminative listening procedures (two sounds judged as same or different). In comparison with age peers, the children with SLI made more discrimination errors on the active listening task regardless of stimulus. The really interesting finding, however, concerned the electrophysiological data. Here, the children with SLI also showed inferior levels of response (less MMN), but only for the speech stimuli. Auditory processing of the tone stimuli was normal.

This pattern of group differences on the passive listening task suggests that the presumed central auditory difficulties in this case actually reflected poor representation of the speech sound system, and thus that the perceptual deficits had more to do with language than with audition.

An Information-Processing Alternative

Over the last 20 years there have been significant changes in our understanding of developmental language disorders, and these changes invite us to consider a different sort of alternative explanation for CAPD—one that focuses on the processes that underlie language rather than on language itself. Instead of viewing language impairment as a *specific* disorder, many of us now view this condition as a consequence of deficits in general information processing mechanisms. For children with SLI, language may present the most obvious learning challenges, but attention and memory difficulties extend into nonverbal areas as well (e.g., Im-Bolter, 2003; Johnston & Ellis Weismer, 1983; Mackworth et al., 1973). Thus, in contrast to the audiologists who define CAPD as a deficit that "is not due to higher-order language, cognitive or related factors" (ASHA, 2005a, p. 2), we argue that the difficulties with auditory processing are exactly a direct consequence of those higher-order factors. For us, the auditory nature of the stimuli does not define the problem. Instead we conclude that the auditory processing difficulties are just one manifestation of a broader cognitive processing deficiency which is likely to cause other learning and performance deficits as well.

A report from the U.S. National Institutes of Health (Sevostianov et al., 2002) lends support to this view. The researchers used electrophysiological and imaging data gathered in both passive and active auditory tasks. Eighteen adults heard tones and were told to (1) ignore them, (2) listen for pitch changes in the right ear, or (3) listen for pitch changes in the left ear. There were two findings of note. First, even in the more passive condition, the activated brain regions included areas known to serve the perception of motion and visual-social cues such as eye gaze. Second, in the active listening condition, patterns of brain activation were stronger than in the passive condition, and they extended into widespread regions outside the auditory cortex, regions that "may play a role in attentional processing" (p. 601). These results seem to indicate that performance on this nonverbal discrimination task—exactly the sort of task that is used to test CAPD—reflects nonspecific attentional processes as well as audition.

Objective Science?

Science is always more influenced by beliefs and values than we like to acknowledge. The phrase "best viewed as" in the position statement of the 2004 working group offers a good case in point. The word *best* clearly indicates that the committee has crossed into the gray zone between belief and evidence. Unable to completely prove their view and faced with uncertainty, our audiological colleagues use familiar frameworks and priorities to interpret the data. And, to be honest, I must say the same of myself as a proponent of an alternative view. Even though I have cited two studies that indicate the role of language and attention in auditory perception, I can't prove that this is always the case or that the children referred for CAPD assessment never have discrete, specifically auditory dysfunctions. To some degree, my perspective on CAPD draws on my general cognitivist views of behavior. The fact that all parties to the debate are arguing as much on the basis of values and perspective as on evidence, may explain our 25-year failure to resolve differences.

Does It Matter?

You may be wondering by this point whether any of this matters. If so, your question is a good one. One of the stunning discoveries of our consensus building in 1995 was that regardless of perspective, everyone in the room was pursuing exactly the same two sets of therapeutic strategies—at least in so far as everyday auditory tasks were concerned. First, we were recommending steps to improve auditory signal quality, such as reducing acoustic competition, or boosting the intensity of the signal through preferential seating or assistive devices. Second, we were recommending steps to enhance top-down aspects of perception, such as increasing language knowledge, minimizing demands on attentional capacity, and teaching explicit comprehension monitoring.

The audiologists viewed these top-down steps as compensatory strategies that made use of the connections between audition and other systems. The SLP and psychology folks viewed these steps as dealing directly with the deficit itself. However, these differences in interpretive frameworks did not lead to different treatment decisions. In the absence of treatments that could actually alter the perceptual mechanism, the best that any of us could do was to optimize the functioning of the deficient system, and there was good agreement at a practical level as to how this could be done.

If all that was important was performance on auditory tasks, the debate over the nature of CAPD indeed wouldn't matter. It is when we think about nonauditory functions that the potential costs of a CAPD diagnosis become clear.

Thinking About Child Language

The Potential Costs of a CAPD Diagnosis

As clinicians we do not have the luxury of waiting until all the evidence is in. So, when we are faced with scientific uncertainty, we need to decide which of the positions that might be valid will best serve our client's interests. One way to do this is to weigh the costs and benefits of one perspective versus the other.

Let's compare the consequences of the various views of CAPD. While the audiological perspective acknowledges that the condition leads to academic and language problems, it clearly identifies audition as the focus of treatment. In contrast, while the alternative perspectives do advocate treatments that improve auditory processing, they go beyond this narrow focus to look at other areas that might be affected by a general processing limitation—most notably, expressive language and constructive comprehension. As a clinician, I am concerned that parents, teachers, and other professionals who see the CAPD diagnosis will attend to audition exclusively, whether intended or not, and will miss other equally important areas of difficulty. The potential costs of such tunnel vision could be great.

 For this reason I believe that we serve our clients better if we assume that many, if not most, of the children who are now being diagnosed as CAPD in fact have non-modality-specific cognitive processing problems that manifest themselves in auditory tasks, and elsewhere. At the very least, we can caution parents and professionals that children who have difficulty with auditory processing often have difficulty with other processing tasks, and schedule children with this diagnostic label for a thorough language assessment.❖

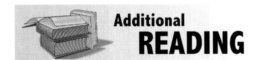

Additional READING

Bishop, D., Carlyon, R., Deeks, J., & Bishop, S. (1999). Auditory temporal processing impairment: Neither necessary nor sufficient for causing language impairment in children. *Journal of Speech, Language, and Hearing Research, 42,* 1295–1310.

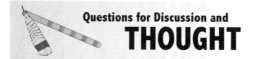

Questions for Discussion and
THOUGHT

1. If the general information processing view of CAPD is valid, what specific sorts of expressive language difficulties could be expected?

2. Why is it primarily school-age children who are referred for CAPD?

3. What values may be influencing the debates about CAPD?

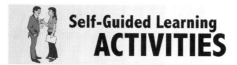

Self-Guided Learning
ACTIVITIES

Make an appointment with an audiologist in your community who regularly tests for central auditory processing disorder. Go over the test battery with him or her. Better still, ask to actually take some of the tests and discuss the diagnostic criteria that are used. Have the audiologist also comment on any therapy recommendations that would follow directly from the test battery. Following your appointment, list the tasks in the CAPD assessment and decide whether they require language, selective attention, and/or working memory.

13 Listen Up!

This essay is about a boy, singing lessons, computer games, and 3 × 10 inch cards. I am not sure, but I think they all fit together. Let's start with the boy. Jay is a nine-year-old with a classic, and profound, language disorder. When first seen by an SLP at age 5;6, he seldom spoke and used only one- to two-word utterances. The initial assessment report noted that "in the classroom he acts as though he were deaf." After four years of intervention, Jay had learned much about language and could express complex ideas relatively well, although his utterances were often ungrammatical. Against the odds, he continued to score above the mean on non-verbal intelligence tests, performed at grade level in math, and clearly enjoyed school. But interestingly, now his friends were saying, "Sometimes we think he is deaf."

In the fall semester of grade 4, Jay's SLP tested his comprehension of spoken text by reading short paragraphs and asking him questions about the content. He was unable to answer most of the questions, scoring somewhere around -5 *SD*. Now comes the interesting part. One week later, when he again met with the SLP, Jay asked to repeat the comprehension test. He knew he had done poorly the first time, and said, "I know how to do it now. I have to listen really hard." His second score was not much better than the first, but his assessment of the problem was right on target.

What do we do when we listen? I don't know of anyone who can explain volitional attention, but that is what listening is. When we listen, we pay attention to a particular auditory signal, having decided to focus on that part of our sensory experience. Not our tired muscles, our growling stomach, or the picture on the wall, but the spatter of raindrops. Try it, right now. Stop reading for a moment and tune in to the sounds in the room. What do you hear?

When you stopped reading and began listening you did at least two things. You instructed your inner attentional mechanism to prioritize auditory information, and you drew on prior knowledge to interpret the sounds that were occurring. Jay most probably has difficulty with both of these mental tasks. The good news is that both of them are amenable to intervention. We know that language intervention provides children with new knowledge that can be used to interpret speech. Intervention may also improve their auditory attention, and here's where the singing lessons come in.

While I was in graduate school, I studied vocal music quite seriously, performing with a small chorale and taking private lessons. During those eight years, something happened to my head. Having invested much time and effort in creating and interpreting musical sound, I became unable to ignore it. For me, background music no longer exists; music is always in the foreground. Although I can't prove it, I believe that my singing experience changed my listening habits (i.e., my attentional priorities). Interestingly, that would also be one way of talking about the putative effects of Fast ForWord® (Scientific Learning Corporation, 1997–2005), the computerized language intervention program that uses acoustically altered speech to try to shape perception.

Preliminary Studies of Fast ForWord

Fast ForWord (FFW) is one of a family of computer-based intervention programs marketed by Scientific Learning. In this program, children practice listening to and interpreting sounds, words, and sentences that are graded in difficulty. The massed-practice training is achieved through attractive computer games that are designed to help children stick with a challenging task. The unique feature of FFW is that the language stimuli have been acoustically altered by increasing the overall duration of the speech and selectively amplifying the fast, transitional elements. The degree of acoustic modification is systematically reduced as children progress through the program. Two outcome studies of FFW have been reported by Scientific Learning personnel and seem to indicate that the program is effective (Merzenich et al., 1996; Tallal et al., 1996). Design flaws make this conclusion premature, but even if it is confirmed, the research does not yet indicate which aspects of the program are important nor why it works (Gillam, 1999).

In 2002, Ron Gillam, Diane Frome Loeb, and Sandi Friel-Patti began a large-scale clinical trial of FFW. In preparation for this project, they conducted five pilot studies, with fascinating results. I will summarize three of them here. Frome Loeb et al. (2001) compared language performance before and after completion of FFW for four children, ages 6 to 8. The assessments were done by graduate students who did not know the purpose of the study, and the battery included spontaneous language sampling in addition to a wide range of standardized tests. The researchers found positive changes on about 30 percent of the measures. However, the gains were much smaller than had been reported by Merzerich et al. and only 10 percent of the measures maintained improvement three months later. Moreover, even though parents expressed general satisfaction with the FFW program, comparison of the pre- and postintervention parental reports indicated that they were seeing no actual changes in language behavior.

Gillam and his colleagues (Gillam, Crofford, et al., 2001) compared the FFW program to off-the-shelf language training software published by Laureate Learning Systems (LLS). Four children participated, two in each condition. As a nice additional touch, two of the children were identical twins, one in each program. After four weeks of treatment (two hours daily), language scores for all four children had improved significantly. This was true for measures derived from spontaneous language as well as from standardized tests. But note that the children who used the LLS software did just as well as the children using FFW. As the researchers comment, "the similarity of the treatment effects...was surprising since FFW and the LLS programs targeted different levels of language, used different types of auditory stimuli, and were designed to promote different kinds of learning" (p. 231).

The FFW games make use of acoustically modified speech, and train children to make subtle perceptual distinctions at the phonetic and syllabic level. Although current marketing of the program barely alludes to this feature, at the time that FFW was first published, manipulation of speech acoustics was considered to be an important reason for its success (Tallal et al., 1996). The LLS games, on the other hand, include no acoustic manipulation and do not provide discrimination drills at the phoneme or syllable level. This and other findings led the researchers to conclude that the observed gains were not due to improvements in temporal processing (Gillam, Frome Loeb, et al., 2001).

Further support for this conclusion came from a backward masking experiment that included the four children from the intervention pilot (Marler et al., 2001). Three of these children showed an initial temporal processing deficit on the masking task, and two of them did show perceptual improvement following intervention. However, much of the improvement occurred after only one week, and error patterns suggested that memory or attention, rather than temporal processing, may have been responsible. Moreover, equivalent improvement was seen for both the FFW and LLS programs. Together these facts suggest that while the FFW program may be effective, the reasons for language improvement may be different than its creators believe.

These pilot study results need replication and the results of the clinical trial will be important. The pilot data do seem to indicate however, that "[both of] these programs promoted attention, encouraged children to respond quickly, and facilitated listening skills" (Gillam, Frome Loeb, et al., 2001, p. 272). This may be problematic news for the company that markets FFW, but it is good news for us because it means that: (1) specialized technology is not the key to remediating language disorders, and (2) it is possible to help children become more successful listeners.

Learning to Listen

Language comprehension requires listening. That may sound simplistic, but I think that as SLPs we have slighted this fact. We have thought a great deal about auditory perceptual processes or about language knowledge, and not enough about the volitional mental focus and selectivity that is implicit in auditory attention. Children normally develop selective listening skills in late infancy, but lags in neural maturation, perceptual deficits, or language delays may hinder this achievement. Children who don't talk get much less practice in listening. If they find the auditory world confusing they may even choose not to listen. Imagine the number of hours a normally developing preschooler spends listening—to playmates, to family, to books, to television. Then imagine the very different experience of a five-year-old who is a social isolate and seldom talks with anyone. Jay now knows that he needs to listen really hard, but he may still lack the ability to do so. My adult experience with voice lessons, and less trivially, the pilot studies summarized above, suggest that it is not too late for him to learn.

Here's where the 3 × 10 cards come in. When I first began my practice, there was a therapy device called a Language Master. This is an audiorecorder that reads tape strips embedded in 3 × 10 cards. A brief message can be recorded on these cards and they can be reused. Jay's SLP has resurrected the Language Master in her closet and has prepared materials for him to practice listening to. With familiar vocabulary and syntax, the emphasis is on language performance, not acquisition. The tasks are organized such that Jay can judge for himself whether he has listened well and understood the message. Once Jay is consistently successful on a set of items, the listening environment can be made more challenging by reducing the volume, or introducing small doses of noise and distraction. Those of you without access to old machines may need to rely on computers to get the same job done, but the idea can remain the same.

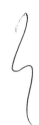

I am not arguing that auditory perceptual processes are unimportant, they obviously are. Nor am I arguing that Jay doesn't need to acquire new language forms and discourse schemes. He does, and each new acquisition will improve his resources for comprehending language. But good old-fashioned listening is something different from either of these, and I thank Jay for reminding me of this.❖

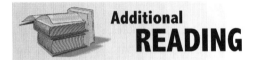

Additional READING

Ruff, H., & Capozzoli, M. (2003). Development of attention and distractibility in the first four years of life. *Developmental Psychology, 39*, 877–890.

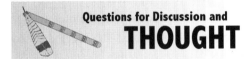

Questions for Discussion and THOUGHT

1. What would make an utterance easier to pay attention to? Does the answer to this question depend on the age, cognitive, or language level of the child?

2. What do the FFW and LLS programs have in common that could account for the improvement seen with both sets of materials? Gillam argues that both of them promoted selective attention. How?

3. What is the difference, if any, between listening to language and comprehending language? What do teachers mean when they say a child "doesn't listen"?

Self-Guided Learning
ACTIVITIES

1. Select short passages from the social science textbook used by a child on your caseload and prepare questions on the content. Focus on material that will be useful in an upcoming classroom lesson. Vary the length of the paragraphs and the complexity of the sentences so that you have several easy paragraphs and several that are more difficult. Keep the child's language level in mind as you select the texts. Have the child listen while you read the set of paragraphs and then answer the questions. Repeat the items three to five times, keeping track of the number of errors and their nature. Does the child's success rate improve? Does the nature of the errors change? What does this suggest about the nature of listening?

2. Visit the Scientific Learning website (www.scilearn.com), the company that markets FFW. What are the strengths and weaknesses of the materials that are presented to demonstrate the value of this program?

Issues in Assessment

Language intervention assumes some sort of assessment—of a community, an environment, or a child. Many times, perhaps even most of the time, we determine with five minutes of observation whether a child's language development meets age expectations. We then spend the next hour(s) administering tests that do little more than add credibility to this judgment.

The essays in this section are about the other times and the other questions. How can we determine what the child knows about the language system? How do we differentiate normal second-language (L2) delays from those that are due to impairment? Why is this child's language delayed? As you read these essays you'll see that I am a bit of an iconoclast when it comes to assessment. I seldom find a reason to test, and have my doubts about the whole differential diagnosis enterprise. Tests don't need advocates. They are so well entrenched in practice patterns that virtually nothing can dislodge them. Language sample analysis (LSA), on the other hand, is less familiar to many SLPs and requires time and expertise. Since I am totally convinced about the value of analyzing the child's everyday talk, these essays contain much about language samples and very little about tests. I argue for the special utility of LSA for charting progress and evaluating bilingual speakers, and suggest ways to streamline the process. You needn't agree with me about tests, but I hope the essays will encourage you to use language sample analysis more often.

14 Fact, Fashion, and Funding Systems

Several years ago, I volunteered to teach a course called Communication Disorders in Special Populations. My students were quick to point out the irony in this assignment given my strong belief that decisions about language intervention do not depend on traditional differential diagnosis. Together we took the opportunity to explore other possible values of diagnostic labels. I won't pretend to cover all facets of this topic in a short essay, but here is some of what we learned.

Fact: The Limitations of Diagnostic Schemes

Differential diagnosis is the task of determining the nature of the condition that has led to a child's language problems, using categories such as retardation/developmental delay, deafness/hearing impairment, autism/autism spectrum, and developmental language disorder/specific language impairment. (Each label following a slash is the more modern term.) These categories are traditionally treated as if they are explanatory and, as SLPs and educators, we often argue that a child's language delay stems from the retardation, the autism, or the language impairment. A quick look behind the scenes, however, indicates the huge fallacy in such reasoning. The fact is that with the exception of deafness, the traditional categories of differential diagnosis are merely labels for clusters of behavior and require no evidence of a causal agent. It is actually quite circular to use the diagnostic category to explain the behavior that was used to establish membership in the category in the first place. Take autism, for example. Since one of the three major criteria for diagnosing autism is language delay, it makes little sense to argue that the language delay is due to autism. I think we have tolerated this lapse of logic in the belief that these categories are somehow isomorphic with those that would emerge if we did have direct causal evidence. Data from a large-sample longitudinal study directed by Isabel Rapin, a pediatric neurologist at the Einstein School of Medicine, invite us to reexamine this faith (Rapin, 1996).

Beginning in the mid-1980s, Rapin and a large team of coinvestigators in six U.S. centers conducted an ambitious test of the validity of diagnostic labels in communication disorders. In line with her training as a physician, Rapin wanted to validate the traditional diagnostic scheme for developmental disorders of higher cognitive function. The research strategy was essentially to collect measures of language, cognitive, and social function, then use sophisticated statistical analyses of the various scores to determine the characteristics that were unique to each diagnostic group. The team made clinical assessments of some 550 children aged 3 to 5. Participants had been selected on the basis of prior diagnoses of autism (high functioning, N = 51; low functioning, N = 110), developmental delay (N = 110), and developmental language disorder (i.e., specific language impairment; N = 270). None of the children had frank neural pathology or significant motor or sensory disabilities. The assessment battery included standardized language tests (TELD or SICD, PPVT, EOWPVT, Vineland), analysis of a spontaneous language sample, extensive cognitive testing, and analysis of a spontaneous play sample. I was asked to serve on the advisory board for this project and so met with the team at least once a year over a period of five years or so.

The findings from this project were published in a 1996 book entitled *Preschool Children with Inadequate Communication* (Rapin, 1996). The researchers did find a few group differences on the various language measures, as follows:

- In the language samples, the DLD (SLI) children were more conversationally responsive, more likely to maintain topic, and less likely to make errors in lexical selection than children in other groups.

- In the test score profiles, children with autism had a peak for expressive vocabulary and a dip for rapid recall of words in a category, whereas profiles for other groups were flat.

Beyond this, however, group differences were seen only in the severity of the delay: low functioning autism < developmental delay < high functioning autism < developmental language disorder. The investigators ultimately concluded that "groups represent very broad and heterogeneous groups and, furthermore, that considerable overlap exists between groups. Social and communication difficulties exist in the DLD [developmental language delay] and NALIQ [developmental delay] groups, language disorders in the NALIQ and AD [autistic] children, and retardation in the AD children" (Rapin et al., 1996, p. 216).

These group findings indicate a clear limitation in the traditional diagnostic scheme: there were very few qualitative differences in the language patterns of children in the various groups, and the signature characteristics of one group actually were seen in other groups as well. Further indication of system inadequacies came from statistical analysis of the scores earned by individual children. Approximately 15 percent of them had a greater than 50 percent chance of belonging to a group other than the one in which they had been diagnosed.

None of these factual findings reflects poor clinical appraisal. My time with the team left me certain that the data had been collected and analyzed in an expert manner. As I listened to the team members talk, and later as I read the monograph, I was reminded of my own participation as a clinician in a similar project conducted in the 1960s at Stanford University. Researchers there had likewise attempted to link our diagnostic judgments to clusters of empirical fact, and had failed (Rosenthal et al., 1972). I remember thinking at the time that they had just not been able to quantify the crucial clinical judgments, but now I wonder if perhaps it is the enterprise itself that is flawed. There may just be too many links in the causal chain between the primary physical agents and the observable behaviors. Put differently, any given behavior can occur for too many reasons.

The practical implication of these research facts seems quite straightforward. If all you know is that a child has been diagnosed as autistic, developmentally delayed, or specifically language impaired, you can make very few predictions about the nature of the child's language. Why, then, do we spend so much time in differential diagnosis? This question leads us to social realities and ultimately to fashion.

Fashion: Diagnostic Categories as Social Constructs

An article in *Time* magazine of January 20, 2003, provided some historical notes on differential diagnosis. The first official attempt to measure the prevalence of mental problems in the United States came in 1840 when the census included a category called "idiocy/insanity." Diagnostic categories proliferated quickly, and in an attempt to create some consistency in their use, the American Psychiatric Association published its first edition of the *Diagnostic and Statistical Manual of Mental Disorders (DSM)* in 1952. There have now been four editions of the *DSM*, and a fifth is being prepared. This diagnostic scheme—a piece of which we use in clinical assessments—tries for systematicity and evidence, but the *Time* writer concludes, "many forces besides science shape it, including politics, fashion, and tradition" (Cloud, 2003, p. 103).

The broadening of the *DSM* criteria for autism over the last 15 years certainly provides one example of the influence of politics and fashion. Many of the children who were once diagnosed as having specific language impairments (developmental aphasia, or the like) are now being diagnosed as autistic. From a scientific point of view, this change has dramatically increased the heterogeneity of the group of

101

persons diagnosed as autistic and has created a problematic discontinuity in the research literature. However, these negative consequences seem to have been overridden by the public appeal of autism. Movies, radio interviews, and popular books about autism arrive on the scene with some regularity, and we speculate about famous historical figures who may have been autistic. To my knowledge there has never been a movie, a radio interview, or an autobiographical account of SLI, and the only public figure I know of to be speculatively diagnosed with this condition is Jean Chrétien, the former Prime Minister of Canada, who is reported to have difficulty with both of Canada's official languages (Teitel, 2003).

It is difficult for professionals to understand why some parents would rather have a child who is called autistic than one who is called language impaired. This may reflect a gap between the popular view of SLI and the parents' everyday view of their children. SLI has long been viewed as a condition that is transient and affects only the speech of young children. Moreover, as a category defined principally by exclusion, SLI is a label that users have never pretended they can explain. Such a condition doesn't fit the experience of parents who know that their affected children have widespread learning difficulties that last well into the school years, and who see the social consequences of early language impairments. They may well find autism a more satisfying diagnosis, particularly now with the autism spectrum option. The autism label is a better fit for what they see in their children, and provides them with at least part of what they are looking for: explanation (albeit illusory); relief; increased tolerance; access to support groups and information; and a sense of shared experience.

However, the label does not yet determine intervention strategies, and the cost of any label may be considerable: stigmatization, stereotyping, false expectations (both high and low), learned helplessness, and reduced access to service. After extensive interviews and focus groups with young adults who had learning difficulties, one team concluded that "many participants in our research were substantially worse off as a direct result of receiving a diagnosis" (Gillman et al., 2000, p. 406). These researchers go on to suggest that professionals should adopt an ethical framework in which the "safety" of a diagnosis is measured by "its value in opening doors and creating opportunities" (p. 407) and should resist diagnostic practices that will restrict opportunity.

Funding Systems and Social Justice

Despite these very real indications of limited value and negative consequences, it seems to me that there is at least one important reason for continuing the business of early differential diagnosis—justice requires it. If health and education benefits for young children are to be offered to the public in a fair and evenhanded manner, there must be a principled system for specifying the persons for whom they are intended. Without a general descriptive taxonomy, the provision of service would be ad hoc, relying on the local administrator's ingenuity, budget, compassion, and longevity.

This is not to argue that public programs need to maintain traditional diagnostic categories such as autism or SLI. At the least, functional criteria such as severity of impairment should be added to these etiologically oriented groupings. Better still, program management could rely on taxonomies that are descriptive instead of explanatory (e.g., that refer to degree of delay without reference to cause). In the final analysis, though, however much we may dislike them, and however far they may fall short of providing real explanations and guidance, diagnostic categories are necessary for legal and institutional purposes. This being true, we must think carefully about how to live with them.

Shared Wisdom

The students in my class tackled this problem with notable success. Here is what they advised after extensive discussion and debate:

- Resist the temptations of certainty; think of the diagnosis as a starting point, not an ending point.

- Remember that a child's "problems" are defined by society's expectations as much as by the child's capabilities.

- Don't be bound by tradition in your own organization of service. For example, try forming a parent group based on the developmental level of the children rather than the reason for their learning difficulties.

- In counseling families and teachers, emphasize treatment strategies and programs rather than explanations. Acknowledge the human desire to name and understand, but move as quickly as possible to talk about learning and growth.

- Give families information about websites that have good quality information.

- Be sure to explore the validity of a label's implications for a given child. For example, some autistic persons are quite social, and some SLI children have serious social difficulties.

Final words on this topic were provided by one student who offered a quotation from the Tao Te Ching. I don't know if we should be sobered or comforted by this evidence that our concerns about diagnosis are a very old story:

> *When you have names and forms, Know that they are provisional.*
> *When you have institutions, Know where their function should end.*
> *Knowing when to stop, You can avoid the danger.*
> *—Lao-Tzu, 520❖*

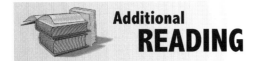

Additional
READING

Weiss, A., Tomblin, J. B., & Robin, D. (1994). Language disorders. In J. B. Tomblin, H. Morris & D. Spriestersbach (Eds.), *Diagnosis in speech-language pathology* (pp. 99–134) San Diego: Singular.

Vig, S., & Jedrysek, E. (1999). Autistic features in young children with significant cognitive impairment: Autism or mental retardation? *Journal of Autism & Developmental Disorders, 29,* 235–248.

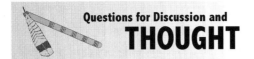

Questions for Discussion and
THOUGHT

1. What sort of experiment would test the validity of the idea that developmental problems are defined as much by social expectation as by the child's capabilities?

2. I argue in this essay that clusters of observable behavior may identify groups of children, but don't provide any real explanation for developmental problems. What sort of information would be explanatory?

3. What is the consequence of redefining a diagnostic category? Take autism versus autism spectrum disorder as an example. How does this change in definition affect your consultation with parents and teachers? Your reading of the literature? Your prognosis?

4. What would be the pros and cons of a workplace policy to the effect that SLPs would not engage in differential diagnosis? What could be done instead?

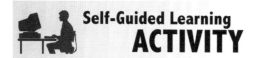

Self-Guided Learning
ACTIVITY

Choose one diagnostic category (e.g., autism, learning disability, SLI, developmental delay) and search the Internet to find information about its speech and language correlates. Spend one hour on this task. When you have finished, make a list of five important things that parents should keep in mind when they consult this computer resource. Prepare a handout.

Be sure to familiarize yourself with the website ratings provided by Tufts University (www.cfw.tufts.edu) and to read their criteria for evaluating online information.

15 Diagnostic Categories and Public Policy

All kinds of images come to mind when I think about political advisors—Royal Commissions, Town Hall meetings, spin doctors, pollsters, Rasputin, Wormtongue. It's actually not clear to me how political decisions get made, but I suspect that the day-to-day reality is more mundane than my images would suggest. Civil servants and assistants to the assistant ministers probably gather opinion, do as much library research as time permits, and prepare position papers which then fuel discussions and decisions on public policy.

Three recent papers should be on the must-read list for these policy assistants. They concern the relationship between autism spectrum disorder (ASD) and specific language impairment (SLI). Right now, government policy in British Columbia provides relatively generous funding to support treatment for children with autism regardless of the severity of their developmental delays. It provides little or no funding for children with specific language impairments. This creates situations in which a child with autism who is doing well in school and has minimal language delay is seen by the local SLP, while the second grader with SLI who speaks like a four-year-old and is not reading, receives very little SLP service.

The policy makes no sense given what we now know about the long-term prognosis for children with SLI and the growing evidence of a continuum or overlap between the ASD and SLI diagnostic groups.

Cortex Asymmetry in ASD and SLI

A research team at Massachusetts General Hospital has published a study of brain volume in children age 6 to 13 years (De Fosse et al., 2004). There were four groups of participants: children with autism and language impairment (ALI), children with autism but no language impairment (ANL), children with SLI, and children with normal language development (NL). All participants were boys and were right-handed. None had evidence of frank neurological damage (e.g., cerebral palsy). Language status was determined with the CELF and with a nonsense-word repetition task. Those considered impaired scored more than one standard deviation below the mean on one or the other measure. Four of the nine boys in the SLI group did not actually meet this criterion, but did have histories of serious language delay.

Sophisticated MRI imaging techniques were used to establish the volume of cortex in regions associated with language (i.e., Broca's area and the planum temporale). There were no group differences in the overall volume of the language regions for each hemisphere treated separately. However, when the researchers compared the relative size of these regions in the right versus the left hemispheres, things got more interesting. A symmetry index was calculated for each child. It turned out that children in both of the groups with language impairment had greater brain volume in the right side Broca's area than in the left side, while children in both groups with normal language showed exactly the opposite pattern. There were no significant differences in the symmetry index between the two language-impaired groups or between the two language-normal groups. Finally, neighboring brain regions did not show significant group differences, nor did the other targeted language region, the planum temporale.

There had been earlier reports of reversed asymmetry in Broca's area occurring in groups of either ASD or SLI children. What is new and important about this study is that the autistic children were divided a priori into those who had language impairment and those who did not, and then were directly compared to children with SLI. This design allowed the research team to conclude that "the volumetric asymmetry...is more closely related to language impairment than to the autism diagnosis" (DeFosse et al., 2004, p. 762), and further, that there may be "a common neurobiological basis of language impairment in autism and SLI" (p. 764).

What Is Language and Language Impairment?

You may have been surprised to read that the participants in this study included a group of autistic children who did not have language impairments. To understand how this is possible, we need to be clear about what the authors mean by *language*. One of the researchers on this study was Helen Tager-Flusberg, who has also published a number of studies of language development in autistic children. A recent report from her lab helps us answer this question.

The opening paragraphs of Roberts et al. (2004) distinguish between pragmatic impairments and language impairments, and the authors clearly mean to exclude pragmatic problems from the domain of language impairment proper. This bias reflects their theoretical ties to what I will loosely call "East Coast" linguistics, in recognition of the influence of Chomsky at MIT. There is a very longstanding theoretical debate among linguists in North America as to what sorts of knowledge are included in the grammar of a language. Theorists in the Chomskian tradition argue that only morphology, syntax, and perhaps some aspects of phonology and the lexicon belong in the grammar. This makes sense given their commitment to a genetically specified, or Universal Grammar. Other language scholars, myself included, are less convinced about Universal Grammar and are more willing to include rules of use as a part of the grammar, or at least a part of the domain of language knowledge. This is not a difference in viewpoints that will be reconciled anytime soon.

The important point here is that when Helen and her colleagues at Massachusetts General talk about a common basis for language impairment, they are using the word *language* in this narrower sense to refer primarily to syntax and morphology. They do not report pragmatic measures, but it is reasonable to assume that the autistic children with "no language impairments" nevertheless had difficulties with appropriate language use. However, such difficulties are not the common ground between SLI and ALI that the researchers uncovered.

Tense Marking in Children with Autism

In line with their focus on syntax, Roberts et al. (2004) studied morphology, in particular the verb inflections that often cause difficulties for English-speaking children with SLI. Earlier work (e.g., Kjelgaard & Tager-Flusberg, 2001) had shown that the profile for those children with ASD who had language impairments was very similar to the one reported for children with SLI, namely, relatively standard phonology, moderately impaired vocabulary, and profound deficits in the use of higher-order semantic and syntactic knowledge. Roberts et al. used elicitation probes to investigate morphological competencies in children with ASD more closely, particularly in relationship to vocabulary knowledge. As expected, the children with ASD who had low vocabulary scores had more difficulty providing the tense forms than did children with normal range vocabulary scores. This might only reflect a generalized language delay. However, the correlation between the morphology and vocabulary scores was actually quite modest, suggesting that grammatical morphology was an independent source of difficulty. More research work will be needed to confirm that the developmental delays in morphology exceed those in other language domains, but it seems likely. Since this is a well-documented pattern of language competencies in many children with SLI, confirmation would again point to continuities between the two diagnostic groups.

Use of Context in Language Comprehension

The third study comes from the Oxford researcher Courtney Norbury (2005) and looks at the way that children use earlier parts of a sentence to decide the meaning of a later occurring ambiguous word, for example, *bank* (river or savings), *bow* (weapon or tie), or *bulb* (light or flower). The task was quite simple. Children heard a sentence then saw a picture. They were asked to decide whether the picture went with the sentence or not. The ambiguous word was placed at the end of the sentence, and the preceding content was either biased toward one of the target word meanings, or was neutral. An example will make this clearer. For the word *bank*, a neutral sentence might be "He ran from the bank" and a biased sentence might be "He stole from the bank." The first sentence could apply either to the river or to the folks that keep your checking account, whereas the second sentence makes you think immediately about money.

Norbury measured the speed of the picture decision. Not all of the items contained ambiguities. But for those that did, she expected reaction times to be shorter for the biased sentences than for the neutral sentences—*if,* that is, children used the integrated meaning of the whole sentence to help them decide.

The four groups of children who participated in this study were comparable to those in the brain volume study: autistic children with language impairment, autistic children with no language impairment, children with specific language impairment, and typically developing children. The findings again demonstrated the limitations of our diagnostic categories. The two groups with language impairments showed less use of context than the two groups with normal language abilities, and there were no differences between these latter two groups. This outcome did not seem to be the result of differences in language knowledge in any simple sense. The sentence syntax used in the items was extremely simple, and the children independently demonstrated that they knew both meanings for the ambiguous words. What was at stake was the ability to make rapid use of meanings of the whole, and a diagnosis of autism did not predict performance on this aspect of language comprehension. Language status turned out to be more important.

The Common Ground

These three studies point to similarities between children with different clinical diagnoses, autism spectrum disorder and specific language impairment. Children in both of these groups showed a reversed hemispheric asymmetry in the volume of Broca's area, a greater weakness in morphology and syntax than in vocabulary, and difficulty in the use of contextual information to interpret word meanings. This evidence of commonality has crucial implications for public policy and SLP practice.

- **Implication 1—Public Monies for SLI Children.** These studies make it very clear that autism is not a homogeneous category. They also show that SLI children have the same sort of language problems that are seen in some autistic children. Justice would seem to dictate then that we pay less attention to diagnostic labels and more attention to individual profiles when setting our SLP service priorities. Some of the children labeled as SLI need more service than they currently receive. We need to share this information with our supervisors, with school boards, and with, yes, public policy advisors, and try to change whatever inequities in funding or service patterns may exist.

- **Implication 2—Generic Therapy.** For years I have argued for a generic model of early language intervention, one in which the nature of what we do in therapy does not depend on diagnosis. I usually justify this position by noting the heavy constraints on language learning and teaching. We can't learn language for a child, we can only arrange the input so that she or he will find the learning task easier. This constraint, and hence the fundamental character of language intervention, remains constant as we move from one diagnostic group to the next. The studies described here provide a second rationale for generic intervention. If some children with autism have the same sort of language problems as children with specific language impairments, they should respond to the same types of intervention. This does not, of course, mean that we conduct the same activities with each child on our caseloads, but that the same principles of therapy apply in all cases.

Similarities and Differences Revisited

I had originally intended to round off this essay right here. But the more I thought about the imaging, morphology, and comprehension studies, the more I wondered how much of the putative common ground was due to current diagnostic standards for autism. In the mid-1980s, a number of researchers reported that 50 to 80 percent of children diagnosed as having specific language impairments also showed some symptoms of autism (e.g., Paul & Cohen, 1984; Rapin & Allen, 1987). The *Diagnostic and Statistical Manual of Mental Disorders*–4th Edition (*DSM–IV;*

American Psychiatric Association, 1994) swept these children into the autism spectrum. Perhaps that is the reason for the current reports of commonalities between the two groups? It was raining anyway, so I took myself off to the library to catch up on an old study.

The U.K. Sample

In the early 1970s, a group of British investigators conducted a study in which they directly compared 20 boys with autism and 20 boys with receptive language disorder on a number of cognitive, social, and linguistic variables. The boys in the two groups were originally matched for age (7 to 8), expressive language age (Reynell–E means of 4;1 and 4;5) and nonverbal IQ (WISC Performance means of 91 and 96). The original diagnosis predated the major changes in the *DSM–IV*, and the original statistical analyses showed no overlap between the two groups in language behavior. Since the participants in this study had been recently retested and interviewed at age 23 to 24 (Mawhood et al., 2000), this study could provide some answers to my questions about the common ground. Did these two groups, who had been identified with the older criteria, maintain their distinctive profiles? The findings turned out to be both fascinating and sobering.

Formal and informal measures of language competence showed that both groups continued to have serious delays and difficulties. Vocabulary skills, for example, were at only the 9 to 11 year level. And when it came to word combinations, only 42 percent of the autistic men and 65 percent of the SLI men were generally using full, grammatical sentences. The autistic men were further behind than the SLI men in conversational skills, following instructions, personal event narratives, and understanding plots, but nearly half of the SLI men showed at least moderate levels of difficulty in these areas as well. Moreover, a surprising number of SLI men were now showing odd prosodic patterns and/or lack of verbal expressiveness.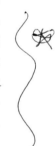

All of the variables were entered into a single statistical analysis to determine whether some combination of strengths and weaknesses would uniquely identify the members of each group. At age 7 to 9, the resulting formula could determine whether a boy was from the SLI or the autistic group with 100 percent accuracy. At age 24 this was no longer possible. Four of the autistic men had made enough progress that their composite scores fell into the SLI range. Unfortunately, 11 of the SLI men had failed to progress or had developed new communication problems that made their assessment profile look similar to the ones found in the autistic group. As the researchers conclude, "although the differentiation seemed clearer in childhood, the two groups appear more similar as they grew older" (Mawhood et al., 2000, p. 556). This particular conclusion was based on assessments of communication and language proficiencies, but similar conclusions were drawn from an accompanying analysis of social competencies as well.

Public Policy Revisited

Admittedly, the 20 boys with SLI in the U.K. sample were not your garden variety preschoolers with moderate expressive language delays. They were primary school children with severe deficits in both expressive and receptive language. The outcomes for SLI children with less severe problems will undoubtedly be more positive. Nevertheless, these findings make it very clear that the recent reports of similarities between autism and SLI in language patterns and in Broca's region asymmetries are not just the reflection of current diagnostic practice. Instead, they do seem to point to a neurobiological common ground that public policymakers have failed to recognize. The difficulties faced by children and youth with serious language impairments are not yet acknowledged in educational funding mechanisms, perhaps because the impairments seem only to involve language. Our government is not the first to underestimate the cost of SLI. The British team notes as well that "educational provision for children in the language group was poorer than for children in the autism group" (p. 555). It seems now we all must learn how to use the growing scientific evidence to change this misunderstanding. ❖

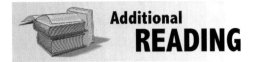

Additional
READING

Kanner, L. (1971). Follow-up study of eleven autistic children originally reported in 1943. *Journal of Autism and Childhood Schizophrenia, 1,* 119–145.

Rapin, I., & Dunn, M. (2003). Update on the language disorders of persons on the autistic spectrum, *Brain and Development, 25,* 166–172.

Wing, L. (1993). The definition and prevalence of autism: A review. *European Child and Adolescent Psychiatry, 2*, 61–74. Available online (www.mugsy.org/wing.htm); discusses various diagnostic criteria used prior to those used currently.

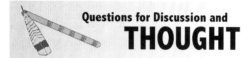

Questions for Discussion and
THOUGHT

1. How does language therapy for a child with autism differ from therapy for a child with SLI at the same age and language level? Why? Does it need to?

2. The next version of the *DSM* may characterize the autism spectrum more narrowly. What would be the consequence for children in your school or clinic?

3. It would appear that there is at least one group of children who could be diagnosed as either SLI or autistic. Discuss the pros and cons of making this diagnosis on the basis of availability of service.

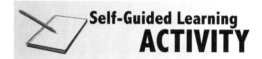

Self-Guided Learning
ACTIVITY

Make a list of all the children with autism you have worked with or observed. Read a description of classic "Kannerian" autism (as in the 1971 article above, or elsewhere). What proportion of the children on your list fit this description?

16 An Old Dog and Two New, Uh, Tricks

Data on the use of MLU in identifying young children with language impairment (Eisenberg et al., 2001) are both encouraging and disturbing. On the positive side, surveys indicate that over 90 percent of the SLPs working with young children now use language sample analysis (LSA) in their assessments. On the not-so-positive side, the analysis often consists of only an MLU calculated from a relatively small number of utterances. Not only is this practice uninformative, it rather misses the point. LSA is not really about numbers, but about description of a child's language knowledge—in detail, and from a developmental perspective.

The power and potential of language sample analysis is only clear when you go beyond MLU to discover what exactly the child does and doesn't know about the structure and use of language. Any numbers generated along with these descriptions can be useful in measuring progress, and can even be translated into normative comparisons with the aid of tools such as the DSS or SALT (Systematic Analysis of Language Transcripts; Miller & Iglesias, 2003–2005). But the real goal of the approach is to describe a child's current language knowledge as it is revealed in real-life communicative talk.

Whether you are among those who only calculate an MLU, or, like me, have been analyzing the details of children's language for decades, there are always new things to learn about the process of language sample analysis. I'm living proof that it *is* possible to teach an old dog new tricks. In this essay I want to tell you about two new tricks that I have learned lately that have made my language sample analyses more reliable and more feasible. The first one is about the numbers, the second about the descriptions that lie beyond.

Trick Number 1: A New MLU

The length of a child's utterances has long been recognized as a valuable index of language competence. But as the child language story unfolded during the 1960s, it turned out that MLU was more than a global index of developmental level. Study after study demonstrated the strong relationships between length of utterance and knowledge of specific language forms.

It is exactly these relationships that make MLU meaningful. Because of them, we can use MLU as a shorthand reference to the grammatical functors, sentence patterns, and words that emerge during the first years of language learning.

Problems with the Traditional MLU

As children learn more about language forms and their use, the implications of MLU values grow less certain. There are two reasons for this change:

- Children have more options for creating utterances of a given length.

- Children's language increasingly reflects properties of the discourse.

Both of these changes represent growth. Children have learned new grammatical patterns and become better conversationalists. However, this very progress creates noise in the relationship between utterance length and the knowledge of specific forms. For example, as children's communication skills improve, they become more able to answer questions. If they are asked many questions, their MLU will be reduced because many utterances will be short answers to these questions (Johnston et al., 1993). The resulting lower MLU value is likely to underestimate their language competence.

The common view among child language scholars is that once MLU reaches 4 to 5, discourse factors render it practically useless as an index of development. This is certainly too radical a conclusion, as is demonstrated by the fact that MLU continues to correlate with age throughout the school years (Leadholm & Miller, 1992). Nevertheless, clinical use of MLU is undoubtedly compromised by the reality of discourse effects.

Fortunately, there is a way to make MLU more reliable at higher levels of development, by using a new calculation procedure. (This new procedure was actually suggested to me by David Ingram in the late 1960s, but is only now beginning to be used with any regularity.) In this alternate method, all imitative utterances, elliptical question responses, and single word *yes/no* responses are removed prior to calculating mean length of utterance. These changes lessen the influence of discourse context.

An Evaluation of MLU2

A few years ago I decided to compare the new MLU calculation method with the traditional one to see how much, and for whom, the MLU values would change (Johnston, 2001). I began with 47 language samples from two groups of preschoolers: 24 normally developing children ages 2 to 4, and 23 children with specific language impairments ages 4 to 6. Samples were collected during play sessions with graduate students. Each sample was 200 to 350 utterances long and included approximately 30 percent narrative material. Two values for mean length of utterance were calculated for each sample, one using Brown's method (MLU) and one using the alternate procedure (MLU2).

To evaluate the new calculation method, I looked at the difference between MLU2 and the traditional MLU expressed as a proportion of the traditional MLU: $(MLU2 - MLU) / MLU$. The results of this evaluation revealed a surprising degree of variability. The proportional difference scores for the 47 samples ranged from 3 to 49 percent, with an average change in *both* groups of 18 percent. For about one quarter of the children, MLU was altered by less than 10 percent, but for another quarter, it was altered by as much as 26 to 49 percent. Not surprisingly, samples in which the adult asked more questions were more affected by the alternate calculation method.

A concrete example may help to clarify the importance of these facts. On average, 28 percent ($SD = 10$) of the utterances in the language samples were responses to questions. Imagine two children who seem to have equivalent degrees of language delay, say MLUs of 4.0 at age 6, but who had interacted with very different conversational partners. Child 1 had been asked few questions, so his MLU2, 4.4, did not differ greatly from the traditional value. Child 2, in contrast, had been asked a very large number of questions, and provided many elliptical answers. His MLU2 was 5.3. Controlling for this discourse variable revealed that the two children, in fact, had quite different language competencies.

Clinical Implications

Implications of these findings for clinical practice are straightforward and important. First, when we use MLU to measure progress in therapy, we need to be sure that the two samples (i.e., pre and post) have equivalent discourse properties. Second, when the proportion of responses to questions is below 18 percent or above 38 percent, we should make some informal mental corrections to our interpretation of the MLU. Low proportions of question responses will lead to overestimation of language competence, and high rates to underestimation. Finally, since the latest version of SALT will calculate both the traditional MLU and a good approximation to MLU2, as well as the proportion of child utterances that are question responses, we can actually explore in some detail the magnitude of any discourse effects.

Trick Number 2: Combining SALT with "The Chart"

The Chart

My second new trick takes us beyond the numbers to the rich descriptions of language competence. But before I can describe the innovation, I need to relate a bit of history. Over 25 years ago, my colleague Mary Sue Ammon and I sat down and organized a number of child language facts into chart form. "The Chart" lists many of the major language forms and patterns that are learned between the ages of 1;0 and 4;6, by order of development. It was intended only as a heuristic organizing tool and was never systematically evaluated. The individual items have each been the object of much study, but establishing their interrelationships was more a matter of by-guess-and-by-golly. Nevertheless, my years of experience with The Chart has convinced me that it is generally valid if used as intended. The Chart is displayed as Table 16.1 on pages 123–124.

Items on The Chart are organized into five levels and three domains (lexicon, grammatical morphology, and highest level sentence patterns). In a sample of 100 utterances we can usually find at least two instances of each grammatical form and sentence pattern that is listed—if the child knows them. Lexical items are more affected by topic and occur less reliably. I usually advise clinicians to tape a sample, transcribe it, and then note on The Chart those forms that do and do not appear. Wherever a form doesn't appear and is at a lower level than other forms that do appear, the clinician must ask whether there were suitable contexts for the missing form. If not, probe tasks can be used to further investigate the child's knowledge. Once item-by-item evaluation is finished, the SLP can identify forms that are next in line, and begin to facilitate their learning.

The Chart makes use of exactly the same research literature that is the basis for other language sample analysis taxonomies (e.g., Lahey, 1988; Miller, 1981; Scarborough, 1990), and any of these sources could be used in the same fashion.

Old Dog, New Trick

Now, back to the innovation. An analysis tool such as The Chart does not address what SLPs see to be the major drawback in language sample analysis, namely, TIME. Transcription is undeniably time consuming and there is no way to reduce this cost except to find someone else to do the transcription (e.g., speech-language assistants, retired English teachers, Rotary club members). However, I have recently discovered a way to dramatically reduce the time required by the analyses themselves. I used the SALT program to assist me in doing an analysis with

Thinking About Child Language

The Chart. I had been meaning to try this for years and finally did. The consequences were astounding. I started with an unfamiliar transcript, and in one hour flat I made normative comparisons for vocabulary diversity, knowledge of relational terms, utterance length, conversational responsiveness, turn length, and fluency; completed a descriptive analysis with The Chart; determined areas for further probes; selected my intervention goals; and wrote a one page summary report.

My strategy was to make lists of the lexemes and grammatical morphemes expected at each Chart Level, then to have SALT find all utterances containing those words or forms and display them in sets by word or form. For example, *because* was included in my Level 4 lists and in a nanosecond, I had onscreen the set of utterances containing this word. Not only could I see that indeed this child used the conjunction *because,* I could also easily scan the six utterances in which it occurred and note whether the conjunction joined two full clauses, whether the subordinate clause was preposed, and whether the child seemed to know what *because* meant. The time savings came from the information management capabilities of computers. Unlike me, my friendly PC could remember all of the Level 3 forms at once, search for them simultaneously (without flipping the pages back and forth), and instantly retype the relevant utterances in sets.

SALT is limited to searches that can be linked to the presence (and position) of specific lexemes, but with a little imagination it is possible to search for key sentence patterns despite this limitation. For example, to look for sentential complements such as "He knew when the movie would start," I searched for mental verbs immediately followed by a *wh-* word. To look for DO suppletion in *yes/no* questions, I looked for the allomorphs of DO in sentence-initial position. Search lists for SALT can be saved and reused at will, so we can collect our good search strategies over time.

A Trick for the Future? A Second Look at, uh, "Uh"

Language sample analysis in general, and The Chart in particular, are open-ended procedures, constantly changing as our knowledge base changes. I recently learned a new fact about language use that may soon work its way into my analyses. In any language sample, there are false starts, self-repetitions, reformulations, and fillers that add length to an utterance without participating in its grammatical framework. As methodologies for analyzing spontaneous speech have evolved over the last 40 years, researchers and clinicians have tended to treat this material as extraneous to the assessment of language competence. In SALT transcripts, for example, this material is called a *maze* and is placed within parentheses, so it can be excluded from the calculation of MLU and treated in separate analyses.

A recent article by Clark and Fox Tree (2002) suggests that while we may wish to analyze maze material separately, we shouldn't necessarily dismiss it as extraneous to the sentence under construction. Based on their analysis of four large corpora of adult speech, these researchers propose that the syllables *um* and *uh* are words, rather than mere noises that fill a pause. To support this view, they provide data about contrastiveness, interpretability, control, and conventionality.

It turns out that the two syllables have differentiated significance, with *uh* marking the initiation of a short delay in speaking, and *um* marking a longer delay. These delays may be due to difficulties in finding the right word, preparation for sentence repairs, or indecision about what to say next. The speaker announces the delay so that the listener will understand that the speaker intends to continue and is working on the production problem. Evidence from experiments indicates that adult listeners use these cues to prepare for crucial incoming information, and to make judgments about the speaker's knowledge state. The fact that speakers can reduce or eliminate these signals in more formal speech registers, indicates that they are under speaker control. And finally, the facts that pronunciation of these syllables varies by English dialect, and that the functions are served by entirely different syllables in other languages (both spoken and signed) indicate that they are not merely an emotive expression, but are conventionalized forms within particular language systems.

I know of no developmental research on the topic of filled pauses. But this study reminds me of research done some years ago by Lucille Hess (Hess & Johnston, 1988) on backchannel listener responses. Her work showed that the simple behavior of nodding one's head while listening requires a very high level of metapragmatic understanding. Young listeners, it turns out, don't nod—probably because they do not yet understand the value or necessity of letting the speaker know that they are getting the message. Clark and Fox Tree's (2002) interpretations of their data suggest that we would find similar developmental patterns for *um* and *uh*. Young children may not yet understand the value of indicating to the listener that they are aware of their momentary speech delays and intend to fix them, or may not be able to disengage from the sentence processing in order to give this signal. In either case, they would not be using these syllables at all.

Thinking About Child Language

What interesting data! It certainly invites us to think differently about "filled pauses" and to consider altering our traditional transcription practices. Decisions about whether or not to include *um* and *uh* in MLU calculations may be moot if these signals are not in fact used by young children. On the other hand, if children do produce these signals, they probably should be left standing within the utterance itself rather than isolated within parentheses. Further research will be needed before we can make these decisions.

The Bottom Line

Language sample analysis is a powerful and feasible assessment method for describing the language capabilities of young children. It is also a method that evolves with our own growing knowledge. New tricks may spring from new technology, a bit of creative thinking, or from new information about the acquisition of specific language forms such as *um* or *uh*. The Chart should certainly be viewed as a perpetual work in progress, and one that you are welcome to alter as you continue to learn from the child language literature. Equally important, language sample analysis is itself one of the best guarantees that we will keep learning. As we puzzle over odd utterances and look for the meanings behind the words, we will deepen our understanding of language and language disorders.❖

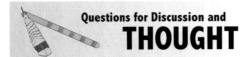

Questions for Discussion and
THOUGHT

1. We've seen that if the child is primarily answering your questions throughout the sample, MLU will be shorter due to ellipsis. What other aspects of the discourse could affect the child's language, and how?

2. Look at the sentence patterns listed on The Chart (see pages 123–124), along with the examples. Discuss any that you do not understand and try to generate further examples.

3. What analysis schemes have you been using to investigate free speech samples? How are they the same or different from The Chart?

4. Choose three grammatical forms from The Chart and discuss how you could quantify performance on those forms. Do the same for three sentence patterns. Do your quantification schemes differ between the grammatical morphemes and the sentence patterns? Why?

Self-Guided Learning
ACTIVITIES

1. **For those new to SALT.** Go to the SALT website (www.languageanalysislab. com) and read the tutorials and case studies. If you are intrigued with the possibilities, approach your local service club to fund purchase of SALT for your team.

2. **For experienced SALT users.** Draw up lists of forms learned at approximately the same time, using The Chart or some other source. Enter these lists into SALT and use them to explore a sample.

Thinking About Child Language

Using "The Chart"

This chart is based on published research from a variety of sources. Since each investigator's methodology, sample, and scoring criteria were different, the overall, composite picture must be treated as an approximation.

Levels. The Chart levels are comparable to the stages suggested in Brown (1973). Note, however, that the MLU values on The Chart are higher than those in Brown and elsewhere. This is because they have been calculated on language samples from which all the question responses have been removed (see Essay 16) and hence are MLU2 values.

Order of Forms. Within each level, groups of forms are broadly ordered by difficulty. All of the forms set off by dashed lines are learned roughly at the same time, and before (or after) other groups of forms appearing above (or below) them. Within these small groups of forms, however, there is no attempt at ordering. Note too that, within a level, there is no necessary correspondence in acquisition difficulty across domains. That is, the first lexical items listed at level 3 are *not* necessarily learned at the same time as the first grammatical morphemes listed at level 3. The only claim regarding equivalences across domains is that all of the items at a level would be expected to emerge during roughly the same period of time. Note that many earlier forms continue in use, and are appropriate, as a child progresses to a new level.

Level of Competence/Performance. Sentence patterns are designated with conventional labels such as N, but this is only meant to describe the surface facts, not the child's mental representations. Forms are listed at the level at which they are used with some reliability—somewhere in between first used and perfectly used. Some may appear earlier in restricted contexts. Note that N = any sort of noun phrase including a pronoun, and this is true also for the N in a PP.

Scope. The sentence patterns and lexical items in the chart are definitely not a comprehensive list, but are merely those which represent significant achievement and/or for which there has been substantial developmental research.

Use. This chart is intended for use in planning clinical and educational programs for children. It is not suitable for research purposes. It is meant to be used as a criteria-referenced checklist, either while observing a given child talk, or while reviewing transcript material. As a rule of thumb, grammatical morphemes and sentence patterns on the chart should appear at least 2 times in a 100 utterance sample if indeed the child knows them.

"The Chart"

Table 16.1 ### Order Of Acquisition for Selected Linguistic Forms

Level/ MLU2	Lexicon	Grammatical Morphology	Highest Sentence Patterns
A 1–1.5	50 words or less, mostly nouns. Comprehension of nouns greater than production.		
B 1.5–2	Some verbs and pivots (e.g., More up, Billy gone). No grammatical forms.		
I 2–3	**here, there, that** **want, wanna** **up, down** (as adverbs) **in, on** (as prepositions) ------- **I, you** ------- **it**	------- plural *s* progressive *ing*	**Sentence with Q intonation** Cookie all gone? **Dem/ quant/ Adj + N** That shoe. Two shoe. Big shoe. **V + N/ Prep Phrase/ Adv** Run fast. Eat apple. Go on top. **N + N/ V/ Adj** Daddy car. Daddy run. Car broken. ------- **"What that?"** (unanalyzed) **"What/Where + N + doing/go?"** (semianalyzed)
II 3–3.5	**this** **What, Where** (in Q) **Why?** (1-word utt.) **me, my**	irregular past tense (a few high frequency)	**V + Modifier + N** Want my dolly. See big dog. **N + V + N/ Prep Phrase** I go in bath. Mommy make cake. **Sentence; Sentence + "too"** I run; Daddy run too. ***Wh* word + Sentence** Where you sit? What Dolly say?
III 3.5–4.5	**with, to, under** **he, she, they, him,** **her, it** **gonna, hafta, gotta** **let's, lemme** ------- **can't, don't** (unanalyzed) **we** ------- **and**	**a, the** possessive *s* copula **is** ------- regular past *ed* 3rd person present *s* auxiliary **is**	**V + N + Prep Phrase** Put the cup on the table. **N + "no"/"not" + V** The man no come. Daddy not play. ------- **Modal/Catenative + V + N** Gonna fix car. Can't put the doggie. **N + V + N + Prep Phrase** John gave toast to the dog. ------- **N + Modal/BE/Catenative + V + N** Mommy is drinking Coke. She can't do it. The boy hafta feed the doggie.

Continued on next page

Thinking About Child Language

Table 16.1—*Cont.*

Level/ MLU2	Lexicon	Grammatical Morphology	Highest Sentence Patterns
IV 4.5-5.5	at, for, by, next to, will, can some, something ------- our, us, their, them, How, Why (in Q) ------- but, if, so, or ------- because other modals (e.g., **should**, **could**) behind, in front of (featured reference obj.)	auxiliary/copula "are", "am" ------- auxiliary **DO** (all forms) ------- auxiliary/copula "was", "were"	**N + V + infinitive complement** He likes to play. The girl wants to go home. **Sentence + 'and + Sentence** We are going to the zoo and we will see tigers. **N + V + Sentence Complement** (includes subject) I saw the elephant eat peanuts. Mommy lets me make Playdoh. ------- **Y/N Question inversion** Is the baby crying? Can Big Bird sing? **...Modal/ BE/ DO + Negative...** I'm not jumping. She won't come. The boy doesn't like it. **N + V + *Wh* complement w/ subject + finite verb** I know where John lives. She said that I could come. ------- **N + V + N + infinitive complement** I want Amanda to play with me. He asked me to go. I told Sam to stop hitting. **Sentence + Subordinate Conjunction + Sentence** My knee hurts because I fell down. I like ice cream if it got chocolate. **DO added in Y/N Questions** Do you know my name? ------- ***Wh* Question w/ aux inversion/ DO added** What are they doing? How can I get up there? Where does that girl live?
V 5.5⁺	nothing, none ------- When (in Q) when (time conjunction) ------- behind, in front of (deictic) before, after, while (conjunctions)	------- auxiliary **HAVE**	**N + V + *Wh* complement w/ infinitive verb** I know what to do. I know how to read. **N + V + complement w/ participial verb** Mr. Byrns saw the boys playing soccer. **...relative clause modifying a Direct Object...** He wants the one that is barking. ------- **Tag Q with auxiliary** She's sad, isn't she? I can go, can't I? **...relative clause modifying a Subject...** The boy who is wearing the red hat is my brother. ------- **N + V + N + *Wh* complement + infinitive** I showed him what to do.

© J. Johnston & M. Ammon (1985) NOTE: PLEASE READ THE EXPLANATORY NOTES (PAGE 122) BEFORE USING.

Thinking About Child Language
© 2006 Thinking Publications.
Duplication permitted for educational use only.

17 Dynamic Assessment

Here's a puzzle for you. Four groups of preschoolers participated in three intervention sessions, each lasting 20 minutes, distributed over a six-week period. They were then retested with a picture-naming vocabulary test and two of the groups showed gains of 8 to 9 percent. That is a surprising degree of success given the modest intervention. What accounted for the change?

My good friend and colleague Ron Gillam at the University of Texas at Austin, was one of the researchers in this study, so I wrote and asked him that question. He in turn talked with his colleague Liz Peña who had also been involved in the study. We exchanged email messages for several days, and I want to share with you what I learned. First though, let's look at the study in more detail.

Fifty-two children participated in this project (Kester et al., 2001). All were attending Head Start preschool programs, played appropriately, and had been judged by their parents and teachers to have normal language development. Most of the children were Hispanic by culture and 65 percent spoke Spanish or were bilingual. The preschoolers participated in three intervention sessions, each lasting 20 minutes, distributed over a six-week period. The intervention sessions were conducted by graduate students, two children at a time. Each pair of children was randomly assigned to one of three treatment programs: Direct Instruction (DI), Mediated Learning Experience (MLE), or Hybrid Instruction (HI). There was also a no-treatment control group. The researchers used a *pretest—teach—posttest* design in order to assess how much the children had learned.

The DI lessons were essentially vocabulary drill, using objects such as a toy chicken. Children were asked to name the objects and were praised for each success. The MLE lessons were drawn from the *Bright Start* curriculum (Haywood et al., 1992), and used scaffolding procedures with worksheets. The goals of each session were discussed with the learners, and then, by modeling and questioning, the children were led to name and describe the various animals and shapes on the worksheets. The HI lessons used the same scaffolding approaches, but this time with real-life objects.

Prior to the intervention, and again following it, all participants were given the first 48 items of the EOWPVT–R. Because of culture and language differences, the researchers calculated percentage correct rather than using standardized scoring methods. Children in the HI and MLE groups had an average gain score of 8 to 9 percent (SD = 4 to 5); children in the DI group gained 4 percent; children in the control group showed no change in their scores. Statistical analysis indicated that children in all of the interventions gained more than the control children, but also that children in the MLE and HI groups gained more than children in the DI group. These instructional effects were reliable and accounted for moderately large to large amounts of the differences in gain scores. To be sure, the changes represent only a small number of test items, but they can be presumed to reflect broader changes in expressive vocabulary. ⓟ intervention section.

Dynamic Assessment and Change

For two of the groups then, the researchers found clear gains in test scores. My questions to Ron were these: What had changed? Did the children learn new words during the six-week program? Or did they merely perform better with words they already knew? To say it differently, were the gains due to changes in competence, or performance? These questions lie at the heart of all intervention research and have special importance for dynamic assessment—an approach to language assessment that is receiving much attention these days.

Unlike the more traditional assessments that collect evaluation data at a single point in time, dynamic assessment attempts to evaluate children on the basis of change over two or more points in time—either change in the size of the performance-competence gap, or change in what the child knows. This approach is particularly important when differences in experience may be responsible for lower levels of performance, as is true for children speaking a second language or living in disadvantaged circumstances.

Current discussions of dynamic assessment draw heavily on Vygotsky's notion of the zone of proximal development (ZPD)—both as an assessment phenomenon and as a key element in cognitive growth. Vygotsky was a developmental psychologist who was director of the Moscow Institute of Defectology (I can only assume this loses something in translation) during the 1930s. He held a strongly social view of the origins of mental growth, and argued that innate processes such as attention and perception are restructured as children internalize functions that are initially present only in external social activity (e.g., the exchanges between adult and child). Vygotsky believed that "learning should be matched in some manner with the child's developmental level" (1978, p. 85), a level that was bounded on one side by the child's "independent problem solving," and on the other side by the child's problem solving "under adult guidance or in collaboration with more capable peers" (pp. 85–86). For him, then, a *level* was not a single point but a whole range of performance possibilities he called the *zone of proximal development* (ZPD). Brown and Reeve (1987) suggest "bandwidth of competence" as a modern label for the same idea. Vygotsky believed that interactive teaching-learning "rouses to life, awakens and sets in motion a variety of internal processes of development in the child" (1962, p. 450). For him, the ZPD was an inevitable consequence of the developmental process itself—a process he saw as the gradual internalization of social events.

The ZPD, Mediated Learning, and Dynamic Assessment

Two notions flowing from Vygotskian theory are central to dynamic assessment: the idea that things can be known more and less well, and the idea that adult-child interactions are the basis for later self-guided learning and reasoning. As played out in the current dynamic assessment literature, each of these ideas has inspired its own assessment paradigm, with its own methodology and its own purpose.

Dynamic Assessment as It Measures the Competence-Performance Gap

One sort of dynamic assessment measures the competence-performance gap, which is the difference between what the child could do given full and reliable use of his or her current knowledge, and what he or she usually does. Although we have much yet to learn about the processes involved, child language data suggests that mental representations continue to change after they are acquired. One result of these changes is that forms become increasingly likely to occur when and where they are needed. Researchers characterize these later changes in different ways depending upon their theories and emphasis areas. The connectionists talk about decreases in the level of activation needed to energize a scheme; the memory folks talk about improved access to stored language representations. In the traditional practice of speech therapy, there is the notion of stimulability; and in more recent practice we have the notion of automaticity or mastery learning. What drives all of this theorizing is the observation that the ability to use what we know improves systematically with time, practice, and further learning.

In this sort of dynamic assessment, the clinician's role is to try to transform the child's initial, independent failures into successes by varying the task structure in whatever way leads to the highest level performance. This may involve using a standardized test, then immediately altering the test procedures to see if the child's performance improves with support. In Vygotskian terms, we are identifying the boundaries of the ZPD. Since there is little opportunity for learning in this brief time interval, we clearly are not expecting to see new knowledge. Instead, we are looking for knowledge that is present but not at first evident. We are also looking at the degree and nature of the support required to optimize the child's performance in order to guide our later educational planning.

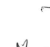

Notice that the direction of mental growth is towards improved, more reliable use, and hence towards a competence-performance gap that diminishes in size over time. Notice too that **the child with a language learning disorder (LLD) might show more difference between the two measurements** than a typically developing child since children with LLD frequently experience performance difficulties due to limitations in working memory and attention.

Dynamic Assessment as It Measures New Schemes

The second sort of dynamic assessment is designed to measure the acquisition of new knowledge. It thus resembles the idea of diagnostic therapy that was popular in the 1960s and is currently reemerging as "Responsiveness-to-Intervention" (Boswell, 2005). If, as in Kester et al. (2001), there is intervention over a period of weeks, followed by a second assessment with the same instrument, it is reasonable to expect evidence of new learning. To the degree that we know the intervention to be effective and know how much learning is typical, we can evaluate whether a child has learning difficulties. Notice that here we would expect **the child with a language learning disorder to show less difference between the two measurements than a typically developing child,** since the typically developing child could be expected to learn more in a given period of time. From a Vygotskian perspective, the long-term goal of teaching interventions is to mediate learning, that is, to create interactions that can be internalized to support and accelerate future learning. In the short term, however, children with language learning disorders should still evidence slower learning patterns.

Dynamic Assessment and the Data

My reading on dynamic assessment left me more knowledgeable about the different goals and procedures within this approach, but at first look, the framework did not seem to fit the Kester et al. (2001) findings. My difficulty was with the nature of the MLE and HI interventions. They didn't seem to be of the sort that should affect test-taking skills, performance with familiar words, or the acquisition of new words. There was no drill to improve access to words the children knew, no talk about tests or practice with test items—only short lessons about squares and triangles and the characteristics of animals.

Further conversation with the authors helped me answer these concerns. The focus of the HI and MLE lessons had been on "special names" for shapes and objects. In the pretest, a number of the children had described the objects that were pictured in the test plates, or had discussed their functions and locations, rather than naming them. At posttest, there was much less of this type of response, and if they didn't know a word, the children would say, for example, "I know it has a special name…it's sort of like *horse*." This suggests that some of the improvement was, after all, due to a new appreciation of what was expected in a vocabulary test (i.e., labels, not descriptions).

Liz Peña also argued that, in fact, the lessons were exactly of the sort that should promote vocabulary learning. From a Vygotskian view, the adult teachers in the MLE and HI sessions may have provided the children with a metastructure for vocabulary learning—the notion that objects had special names. The questions and examples in the adult-child interaction could be internalized by the child and could mediate further learning. Rather than just generally paying attention to adult talk, the children would be primed to listen for new special names (i.e., new labels for object classes). This, in Peña's view, was the second source of the improved test performance in the MLE and HI groups. The intervention not only helped children understand how they should report their old knowledge, it also alerted them to notice, store, and remember any new noun labels they might hear.

Practical Advice and a Promissory Note

I still have questions about these interpretations of the Kester et al. (2001) data. Among other things, the idea of mediated learning seems more suited to reasoning and problem solving than to vocabulary learning. Nevertheless, my reading and thinking about dynamic assessment and the ZPD took me right to the heart of debates about the nature of development. My theoretical commitments do not put environmental influences at the top of the list, and I certainly don't share Vygotsky's view that all mature thought has social origins. I will admit though, that the larger literature on supportive contexts for learning (Brown & Reeve,

1987), as well as results from mediated learning experiments like the one described here, intrigue me enough that I have added it to the list of things to study further.

In the meantime, I think I have learned something valuable about dynamic assessment—namely, that it comes in two flavors, each of which makes a different prediction about the performance of children with learning disabilities:

- **Dynamic assessment done in a single session, with a single body of knowledge assessed and reassessed in different ways with increasing amounts of support.** This sort of DA essentially looks at the performance-competence gap, and, except where socio-cultural factors intervene, the child with LLD can be expected to show the wider gap. Effective use of this strategy requires us to think systematically about types and levels of support.

- **Dynamic assessment done over a period of weeks, with intervention sessions occurring between two administrations of the same measurement tool.** This sort of DA essentially looks at new learning and the child with LLD can be expected to learn less, and thus to show the lesser disparity. Effective use of this strategy requires us to know how much learning to expect from a given program and time frame.❖

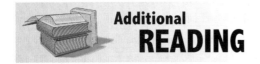 **Additional**
READING

Freeman, L., & Miller, A. (2001). Norm-referenced, criterion-referenced, and dynamic assessment: What exactly is the point? *Educational Psychology in Practice, 17,* 3–16.

Gutierrez-Clellen, V., & Peña, E. (2001). Dynamic assessment of diverse children: A tutorial. *Language, Speech, and Hearing Services in Schools, 32,* 212–224.

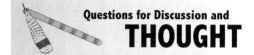

Questions for Discussion and
THOUGHT

1. What are the respective goals of the two types of dynamic assessment? When would you use each in assessing language? With whom?

2. If a child doesn't immediately use a targeted form, how could you vary the situation to find out if the child really knows nothing about it?

3. What are the challenges of interpreting the results of a dynamic assessment?

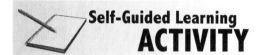

Self-Guided Learning
ACTIVITY

If you are not already using some element of dynamic assessment in your assessment battery, prepare a brief activity that does so. Answer the second discussion question. Then make up a sheet on which you list three to five ways that you can try to elicit a language form that seems to be missing from the child's repertoire (e.g., free play, free play but you provide a high number of examples of the form, structured language game mixing several target forms, etc.). Each of the steps should provide a further increment of support for use of the language form. Make your assessment sheet generic, so that you can use it with any child and any grammatical form that you want to explore during an assessment session. The next time you give a language test to a child, chose an item that the child fails, and try out your dynamic assessment scheme.

18 To Test or Not to Test

That is the question, isn't it? Especially when we are concerned about measuring progress in therapy. Standardized tests play a key role in diagnostic judgments, but have been widely criticized as inappropriate for measuring gains or planning programs. An oft-cited article by McCauley and Swisher (1984), for example, argues that tests are designed to yield general indices of language performance that resist change over time, and moreover, that they lack both the number and variety of items needed to track progress.

Clinicians in Canada apparently have a different view. A research team in Halifax surveyed 144 SLPs regarding their use of standardized language tests (Kerr et al., 2003). For clinicians working in schools, standardized tests ranked #1 for diagnosis *and* for describing a child's language system *and* for goal setting. Tests ranked #2 for measuring progress, falling only a bit behind "observations in context." In all cases tests were preferred over the use of criterion-referenced procedures or language sampling.

This contrast between expert advice and actual practice is puzzling. Not that I think we experts are always right, but in this case the arguments are very close to the facts and hard to refute. Standard scores are inherently stable and tests do have very few items for any given language skill or area of knowledge. As one of my colleagues asked this week, "If tests are such a bad idea, why do smart people continue to use them?" I still cannot answer that question, but two very recent research studies have helped me clarify the issues.

Correlations between Test Scores and Measures of Spontaneous Speech

Condouris et al. (2003) investigated the relationship between test scores and language sample variables in 44 children with autism, ages 4 to 14. The children were verbal, had a group mean performance IQ of 90, and were willing to be tested. The researchers focused on those areas of language where there were tests available, namely vocabulary and grammar. They administered the PPVT–III, the EVT, and portions of the CELF to each child and also taped a 30-minute play session with the child and a parent. A 100-utterance transcript was prepared from this session, and SALT was used to generate mean length of utterance (MLU) and number of different words (NDW) from the sample. The Index of Productive Syntax (IPSyn) was used to quantify the child's grammatical knowledge.

The researchers wanted to know whether the two approaches (i.e., standardized tests and language samples) would provide the same picture of the child's language. In their first set of comparisons, the researchers correlated raw scores from all of the various measures. Both MLU and NDW correlated significantly with performance on tests, and the strongest links occurred where you would expect them—where the test and the language sample variables both focused on grammar, on vocabulary, or on global competence. Correlations with IPSyn were not significant.

Correlations just look at the relative values of scores, not the absolute values. Even if one set of scores put all of the children in the normal range and the other set put them all below -1.5 *SD*, the two sets of scores could be perfectly correlated as long as the children were ranked similarly in each one. Condouris and her team wanted also to compare the absolute value of scores from standardized tests and natural language samples. To do this, they treated the language sample variables in a quasi-normative fashion by using the SALT and IPSyn reference databases. They then looked at the degree of delay that was indicated by tests versus language sampling, child by child. In over half the cases (55 percent), test scores indicated a less severe delay than was indicated by the language sample measures.

The results of this study certainly indicate that tests of grammar and vocabulary tap into the same pool of knowledge that is reflected in language sampling, even for children with autism. This is good to know, but hardly surprising. The findings regarding the severity of delay are more interesting. It could be that children with autism, especially those that are older and verbal, find the structured testing situation conducive to peak performance. Or, it could be that children with autism fail to use the full range of their verbal abilities in spontaneous conversation. If either of these explanations were true, tests would be overestimating the everyday verbal capabilities of children with autism—at least for those who are high functioning and cooperative. This information is useful, but the data for this study were only taken at one time point, so our opening question remains largely unanswered. What about using test scores to measure progress?

Measuring Progress in the Communication Abilities of Young Children with Autism

That brings me to the second study that compares assessment approaches—a thesis project conducted by Susan Fawcett at the University of British Columbia (Fawcett, 2003; Fawcett & Johnston, 2003). The government of British Columbia has been funding an Early Intensive Behavioral Intervention program for young children with autism, and Pat Mirenda, a colleague in the Special Education Department at UBC, has been evaluating this program. As part of her evaluation, Dr. Mirenda and her team gave a battery of standardized tests to half of the 75 children in this program at regular intervals. As it turned out, one of the treatment centers also was making videotapes of therapy and play sessions around the same time as the testing. Both of these data sets were made available to Fawcett so that she could compare the findings from standardized tests with the findings from spontaneous behavior samples for the same children over time.

Twelve children at the center were in the program evaluation sample, but there were only seven who had taping dates that coincided with testing dates, who had clear diagnoses of autism, and whose families consented to participate. For these seven, Fawcett transcribed 30-minute tapes at each of two points in time, either 6, 12, or 18 months apart. After viewing the Time 1 (T1) tapes, she identified three to five areas of behavior that would make good learning goals for each child, and designed a way to measure each. There were goals related to preverbal communication (amount, mode, function), spontaneity (imitative versus nonimitative utterances), relevance (topic maintenance, joint attention), speech sounds (babbling, intelligibility), length and complexity of verbal utterances, and propositional complexity. There was considerable overlap of goals across children, but no two children's goals were exactly the same. The T1 and T2 transcripts were then coded for the pertinent variables, reliability checks were performed, and change scores were calculated.

As the final step in her analysis, Fawcett compared the findings from the standardized tests with the findings from the spontaneous behavior samples. It was challenging to find a way to summarize the seven case studies. Fawcett decided finally to make binary judgments for each measure for each child as to whether or not gain was evident. Child 4, for example, was evaluated in the areas of communication (function, amount, mode), spontaneity, speech sounds, and vocabulary. His rate of communication doubled from T1 to T2. He made no gains in regard to mode of communication, but his vocalizations were more likely to be communicative, and the commenting function appeared. This child's speech sounds did not progress, but there was a modest gain in number of words used, and a large increase in the proportion of appropriate responses. Overall then, five out of seven of the behavior sample variables showed gain. None of the standardized scores from tests showed gains, although parents reported more of the communicative gestures listed on the CDI.

Across all seven children, Fawcett found that the two assessment approaches led to different conclusions about progress in 55 percent of the comparisons. In each of the divergent pairs, it was the behavior sample data that showed gain and the standardized score that did not show gain.

Program Evaluation versus Child Evaluation

In thinking about the results of these two studies, it is important to distinguish between two different types of evaluation—evaluations of programs, and evaluations of children. When we evaluate a program, one of the necessary questions concerns efficacy. Those responsible for funding and policy want to know how much of the observed gain can be attributed to the effects of treatment. The only way to answer this question is through the use of a control group, either one comprised especially for the evaluation, or one implicit in the use of standardized test norms.

In the British Columbia study, government was unwilling to fund a control group and so the evaluators needed to use standardized scores in order to talk about efficacy. There is a worrisome cost to this decision, however. Children who remain nonverbal or uncooperative can show no gains. And even for the verbal children, unless their learning rate accelerates into the supranormal zone, the standard scores will still show no gains.

To ameliorate the extreme conservatism of such findings, Dr. Mirenda has also collected parent report data and will conduct a thorough analysis of the test raw scores. Such data cannot address efficacy, but they may at least document any changes that have occurred. The problem here is that tests are not very sensitive gauges of change. Most language tests have been constructed as general survey measures, with just a few items in each of the many subdomains of language. This means that even the raw scores may fail to reflect the gains that have occurred.

Thinking About Child Language

Now we come to evaluations of children. Many of the questions that motivate our clinical assessments are descriptive (e.g., What does Joey know about communication? Does this child use the auxiliary with more accuracy now?). Simple questions about change do not require a control group. Fawcett's data make it quite clear that if you want to know about a child's use of auxiliary verbs, or a child's use of communicative gesture, naturalistic behavior samples are more likely to provide the information you want. This is true for at least three reasons: (1) because the measures can be designed to focus on particular areas of language, (2) because there are likely to be more opportunities for use and hence greater sensitivity to new knowledge or new levels of performance, and (3) because the child need not be compliant.

Unfortunately, there is a cost to the use of spontaneous behavior samples as well. Without more information about the reliability of the measures we create, it is hard to know if a larger number represents a true gain. And even more importantly, without controls we cannot address efficacy. Our controls may take the form of multiple-baseline measures for a given child or of comparisons between children matched on pertinent characteristics. Both are quite feasible, but they do present challenges in the press of day-to-day clinical activity.

I am going to end this essay with the heretical suggestion that we do not always need to prove efficacy at the level of the individual child. What we do need is a good picture of the child's present knowledge so that we can plan the best possible learning experiences. Tests cannot provide that information. What we also need is evidence of progress so that we can be encouraging to families and clients. Again, because they are less sensitive and more conservative, tests will not give us the best record of growth. On balance, and recognizing that there are costs associated with each assessment approach, I believe that naturalistic behavior sampling gives us the best value for time spent once the initial diagnosis has been made.❖

136

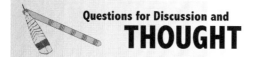

Questions for Discussion and
THOUGHT

1. I conclude that measures of efficacy for individual children are not always needed. Do you agree? When are such measures useful? When not?

2. Is it reasonable to require change in standard scores as proof of efficacy? What does it mean if a child's standard score remains at -1.3 *SD?* Could this fact hide actual improvement? When and how could this happen?

3. Have you ever tried to explain a standard score to parents or family members? What do you tell them to expect in regard to change?

4. Are you convinced by intervention studies that track different goals for each child instead of putting all of the children on the same program? What are the assumptions, strengths, and weaknesses of these individualized designs?

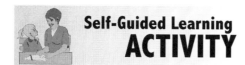

Self-Guided Learning
ACTIVITY

Replicate the Fawcett (2003) study in miniature. Select one child on your caseload for whom you have recent test scores. Transcribe a language (or communication-behavior) sample. Select your intervention targets and create quantified measures for each. These might be, for example, percentage of communicative acts that are verbal, number of utterances in 10 minutes, percentage of utterances with complex sentence structure, percentage of all initiations in a conversation that were made by the child versus adult. Be imaginative. Try to have at least a few areas for which you have both a test score and an informal measure. Put your assessment data in a folder, continue to provide service for six months, then repeat both the tests and the informal measures. Compare the way that each measure does or does not show changes. Pay attention to problems that arise as you try to interpret your data. Read this essay again.

19 "But That's Another Story"

What a curious expression. How can we have this strong sense of what belongs in a particular story? Something in a tale we are telling marches us right up to an interesting fact or event, and then we stop short and choose not to include it, explaining to our listener that it doesn't fit. Or, think about another familiar expression, "It's the same old story." When we say this we're not talking about *The Frog Story* or *Beowolf,* or any particular tale. We're staring right through a specific set of characters, problems, and places, and recognizing well-worn general themes and relationships.

The competencies that allow us to use these two expressions are sophisticated and complex. I would be surprised to hear any school-age child saying either of them, and certainly not a child with developmental language problems. Before children can rule out another story or recognize the same old story they must construct a large number of general event representations, and discover the culturally appropriate properties of a story. Moreover, these *scripts* and *story grammars* must be so familiar and easily deployed that the child's analysis-of-the-moment does not break down from excessive processing load.

It's been more than two decades now since I wrote my first article on the development of narrative discourse (Johnston, 1982b). Notions such as story grammar, script, and cohesion were relatively new then and pointed clinicians toward language units beyond the sentence. It was my sense at the time that the developmental research on narratives had opened up an exciting new opportunity for intervention with school-age children. This has certainly proven true, and we are beginning to understand why.

Narrative as a Predictor of Outcomes

A team of British researchers has been following a large group of children with specific language impairments since they entered special language classrooms at age 7 (Botting et al., 2001). The children were reassessed at age 11 and divided into those with good and those with poor outcomes on a battery of standardized language tests. The battery included tests of lexical comprehension and production, verb morphology (two tests), syntactic comprehension, and word association. *Poor outcome* was operationally defined as having scores that were lower than -1

SD in three or more of these six measures. The initial test battery had included these same areas of language performance, but had additionally included a narrative test, a test of articulation, a nonverbal intelligence scale, and information about family income and maternal education.

The researchers evaluated 117 children at age 11. Of these, 88 (75 percent) fell into the poor-outcome group. All of the test scores and demographic facts from the initial testing were put into a multiple regression analysis to determine which was the best predictor of language outcomes five years later. The answer was narrative, and to a lesser degree, grammatical morphology. For children who scored at the 50th percentile or better on the narrative task at age 7, even if they performed at or below the 10th percentile on morphology, the probability of having a poor outcome was reduced from 75 to 50 percent. Interestingly, maternal education, income, and nonverbal IQ did not emerge as strong predictors once narrative was considered. These variables may have influenced outcomes, but their predictive value was not as great as the narrative scores.

Demand for speech-language services in the schools is increasing and in many places, SLPs are having to make hard decisions about which children to see. The Botting et al. (2001) data on the predictive value of narrative could help with those decisions. Remember, though, that all of the children in that study were receiving language therapy, so we don't know whether the good-outcome group would have done as well without any service at all.

Did you notice that although the strongest predictor of language outcomes in Botting et al. (2001) was a narrative score, the outcome measures did *not* actually include any measure of discourse? Narrative performance at age 7 proved to predict vocabulary, morphology, syntactic comprehension, and word association at age 11. How can this be? I think there are two forces acting in synergy during the school years: grammatical knowledge enabling text, and text knowledge enabling further grammatical development. Children who have had more success in learning words and sentence patterns will be better able to acquire narrative schemes because they are not having to invest as much processing resource at the sentence level. The new narrative schemes, in turn, serve to increase the opportunities to learn new language forms by improving access to classroom discourse and other texts. In contrast, children who are still having difficulty with the basic grammatical forms as they enter school will have had less opportunity to acquire narrative schemes and experience this general enhancement.

Jumping Around and Leaving Out Things

An interesting study by Miranda et al. (1998) illustrates this latter relationship between sentence and text. The researchers asked 8- and 9-year-olds with relatively severe SLI to create five short personal event narratives, using prompts such as, "When I was in second grade, my brother and I got to go to camp. Has anything like that happened for you? Tell me about it." Children in this SLI group were all in special language classrooms, and had scores of -2 *SD* on standardized language tests. Given my earlier explanation, we might expect to find immature narrative forms in these SLI children since their lexical and grammatical capabilities are so delayed. We might also expect to see processing breakdowns as they struggle to do many things at once, none of which they can do well.

The researchers compared narratives from the SLI group to those created by children in two control groups. The first was age-matched and the second group, three years younger, was matched according to scores on the IPSyn, a test of sentence-level productive syntax. The team examined these five dimensions of the narrative texts:

- **Thematic consistency**—Does the child stick to the main story line?

- **Event sequencing**—Does the child order events chronologically, or indicate a choice not to do so?

- **Explicitness** (including reference)—Does the child include everything that a particular listener needs to know in order to follow the story?

- **Cohesion**—Does the child use devices such as anaphoric pronoun and conjunction to tie sentences together?

- **Fluency**—Does the child tell a story without needing to reformulate or repair their utterances?

The comparisons that were particularly telling were the ones with the language-matched, younger children. In some respects, the personal narratives told by children with SLI were similar to, or more advanced than, those of their language peers, namely in length and explicit use of connectives. But most measures indicated that the stories they told were less mature than those told by younger control children at the same language level (as determined by sentence syntax). The children with language impairment included more irrelevant content, skipped over or reordered more key events, left more of the story implicit, and made more reformulations than did the younger controls.

These findings will come as no surprise to clinicians who include narrative tasks in their assessment and intervention sessions—and who have, like me, tried to decipher text such as, "We leave our dogs outside. Every single day. The other dogs come over to our house and play together and got struck. We put in our car and we, we drive him and get out our car and left it there" (Miranda et al., 1998, p. 662). This tale starts reasonably well, but breaks down after "play together." There is certainly a problem with explicitness, cohesion, and perhaps even sequencing.

A Key Assessment Opportunity

The Miranda et al. (1998) data illustrate how difficult it can be to acquire narrative competence when sentence-level grammatical knowledge is delayed. The fact that the younger language-matched controls and the SLI group were at a similar language level is at first puzzling. If there is a connection between sentences and texts, shouldn't these groups have performed more similarly? I think that the solution to this puzzle lies in the fact that basic grammatical learning is asymptotic. There is a finite amount of material to learn and at some point even children with language impairments manage to acquire that knowledge. For normally developing children, the asymptote will occur around age 5 to 6 as they enter kindergarten; for the language-impaired child, some two years later, at age 7 to 8. Note, however, that once children enter the asymptotic zone, there is no way to know, at a single assessment point, how long they have been there. Children who all know the same grammatical forms could easily have known them for varying lengths of time. To speculate a bit, the younger control group in Miranda et al. may have reached the asymptote with ease, and long ago enough to be well into the acquisition of narrative forms. The SLI group, though seemingly at the same level of grammatical knowledge, could have just arrived at that point and done so with enough difficulty that they have had little opportunity to learn about narrative. (See Essay 10 on page 67 for further discussion of this point.)

This account is certainly oversimplified, but it does introduce an important assessment opportunity. If indeed, knowledge of sentence-level syntax becomes a poor index of language growth around the ages of 5 to 6, we need to look elsewhere if we want to make meaningful normative judgments. The shift is clear in standardized language tests where school-age tasks are increasingly oriented toward language performance rather than grammatical knowledge. Our informal assessments need to shift as well, away from checklists of sentence patterns to performance measures such as production breakdowns, and also to descriptions of larger language forms such as narrative.

Data from a recent workshop given by Jon Miller confirm the importance and opportunities of narrative assessment (Miller, 2004). As he reviewed data from the SALT reference data bases, I was fascinated to see a marked plateau in the MLU values obtained from 5- to 6-year-olds *and* an absence of this plateau in a composite narrative measure for the same age group. These data are, of course, exactly what my tale of asymptotic learning would predict since sentence-level grammar is well established but narrative is in a period of rapid development.

Miller also made some valuable comments about the advantages of using narrative material rather than conversational material in normative comparisons of spontaneous language. First, since the language we produce depends in part on what we are talking about, variations in topic can introduce noise into our analyses. Conversational topics emerge and evolve out of largely unplanned social interaction. Narrative topics, on the other hand, can be more closely controlled through the use of the same story material for a narrative retelling, or the same wordless books or pictures to elicit children's own stories. Second, conversations are organized incrementally, turn by turn, while narratives are organized in advance. Since the goals of coherent narrative therefore place an additional processing burden on each sentence, grammatical weaknesses should be seen more quickly. The potential utility of shorter texts is a welcome solution to the transcription problem.

There are now many good reasons to dust off our resource materials on narrative and make plans to incorporate storytelling tasks into our routine assessment activities. It is clear that the narrative task is demanding, and that a child's narrative performance in the primary years is a key index of language proficiency. Narrative measures will also help dissolve illusions of recovery where they exist, and allow us to recognize the service needs of children who are at risk for continuing difficulties with oral language use. It may also prove feasible to collect narratives from all children on our caseloads since they require less of our time than conversational samples.❖

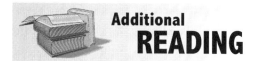

Additional
READING

Johnston, J. (1982b). Narratives: A new look at communication problems in older language disordered children. *Language, Speech, and Hearing Services in Schools, 13,* 65–75.

Trabasso, T., & Van den Broek, P. (1985). Causal thinking and the representation of narrative events. *Journal of Memory and Language, 24,* 612–630.

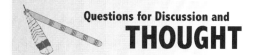

Questions for Discussion and
THOUGHT

1. Each group member should bring a narrative collected from a child on her or his caseload. Take turns reading the narratives to the group. Following each reading, discuss how well the child has done on each of the five dimensions studied in the Miranda et al. project.

2. How could you decide whether a child has reached the point where language performance, rather than the acquisition of new patterns, is the essence of development? (Remember that vocabulary growth is not asymptotic. We continue to acquire new words throughout our lives.)

3. Take two language tests that your group prefers to use for children ages 7 to 9. Look at each subtest; does it measure language knowledge, language performance, or both equally?

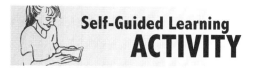

Self-Guided Learning
ACTIVITY

Find a story you could use for a story retelling task. It should have at least two to three episodes and take you at least a minute to read aloud (one episode and less time for preschoolers). You could write one, or take one from a test. Select a child on your caseload (in the 8 to 10 year range, if possible) and ask this child to listen to the story, then retell it. (Motivate the retelling by having the child record a version for you to share with other children, or tell the story to a puppet.) After the session, evaluate the story on each of the five parameters in the Miranda et al. project. Based on this evaluation, alter your story to make it more difficult or less difficult (e.g., more or less familiar vocabulary, more or less complex syntax, more or fewer episodes, more or less familiar events, include a flashback, include mental events, and so on). Repeat the task two weeks later with this revised text. Does the child's performance change?

20 Narrative Schemes and Processes

There's nothing quite like a good story, well told. We use them to teach, to entertain, and to move us out of the real world into the world of gods, heroes, and dreams. They evoke wintry northern nights, campfires, and memories of our favorite storytellers. For SLPs, stories are additionally important because they move children beyond the sentence into larger units of language, and into the challenges of language use in context.

Mental Frameworks That Structure Narratives

Successful narratives are planned texts. The storyteller must create the major theme of the story, organize various events around this theme, and keep it all in mind while formulating the utterances needed to convey the story to a listener. These storage and coordinating tasks may be too much for children whose capacity is already taxed by the task of creating a sentence. The fact that stories can be organized around temporal and causal concepts rather than pure logic means that they carry a lighter processing load than many expository forms (Hudson & Shapiro, 1991). They are, nevertheless, challenging.

Storytellers and listeners alike use mental schemes of two sorts in addition to their basic grammars (Naremore, 1997). First, they employ general event knowledge about the types and order of events that are likely to occur in a particular context (e.g., going to the movies, going hunting, going shopping). These *scripts* begin to develop during the preschool years and are a product of experience, either first hand or derived from books, TV, or movies. Second, they employ *story grammars* of one sort or another to structure the actual telling of the story. These frameworks are again derived from experience, this time with oral stories as well as books and movies, and include ordered slots for information units of specific types. In mainstream North American cultures, a good story is likely to be one that is problem centered; includes attempts and outcomes; and comments about the characters' feelings, motives, and plans.

Story grammars and scripts reside in long-term memory. Whenever a child attempts to compose or understand a story, he or she must call up these schemes from memory and keep them active while filling in the content of the moment. This retrieval of information from long-term storage is usually viewed as one of

145

the important functions of a central executive. The exact mechanisms of this aspect of cognition are not yet understood, and it is likely that more than one mechanism is involved. Be that as it may, there can be little doubt that storytelling entails the planful recall and coordination of highly diverse information, both very particular and very general. Once recalled, these schemes must also be held in mind to guide the storyteller's decisions about what to say next and how to say it. These higher-level processing demands are, of course, in addition to the processing requirements that always occur in language production or comprehension. Children with more effective central executive functions will certainly have an advantage, and children who have both language and working memory deficits will find it particularly difficult to create coherent, cohesive narratives.

Narrative and Working Memory

Two new studies from our Child Language Lab at UBC attest to the value of viewing narrative from a processing perspective. The first (Moser, 2003; Moser & Johnston, 2004) focused on working memory. Twelve children with SLI and a matched group of age peers with normally developing language were given a set of working memory tasks along with a narrative test. Two of the memory tasks were auditory-verbal and two were visual-spatial. In each mode there was an easier storage-only task and a more difficult storage-plus-processing task. In the auditory mode, for example, the storage-only task was similar to the traditional digit-span task (i.e., children were required to repeat a series of lists of familiar nouns). In the storage-plus-processing task, children again heard lists of nouns and were required to repeat them. First, however, they had to reorganize the words according to the size of the referent, so that they repeated all of the words with small referents together and all of the words with large referents together. For example, children heard the list *car, watch, dog, ring,* then reordered them to *watch* and *ring, car* and *dog*. Children in the SLI group scored lower than their age peers in the auditory-verbal tasks, particularly in the one that required reorganization of the words.

In order to look at possible associations between working memory and narrative, Moser used two scores from the Test of Narrative Language (TNL), the composite production score and the score for the story that is self-generated from a single picture, the most difficult storytelling task. There were significant and moderately strong correlations between both of these scores and the working memory span earned on the auditory-storage-plus-processing task. Although less strong, there was also some indication of a relationship between the visual working memory span and narrative. This raises the interesting possibility that the crucial aspects of working memory are quite general and modality free.

The second study (Curan et al., 2004) explored the processing demands inherent in narrative texts by looking at the relationships between grammaticality and coherence. We again used two subtests from the TNL, the self-generated stories from the five-picture sequence and from the single picture. In the Moser (2003) study, the TNL had clearly differentiated the group of SLI children from the age-matched control group with normal language development. Mean score for the three narrative production tasks was 32.8 for the SLI children versus 52.2 for the controls. However, as we scored those stories, we noticed that the same score could be earned for very different reasons. Here are two stories that both earned a score of 14 in the single picture task.

Story 1. They walked to a camp place where there aliens with six legs.

Her brother said, "No!"

"Don't go, they're aliens with six legs."

"That dog's not even real."

"And they spot on their head."

"There's alien in there."

"They're gonna be here forever."

That's what he said to the boy.

They're waving to people.

And she said, "There's spots on the people's legs."

The alien ship says nothing.

But we can't read it 'cause it's in alien words.

And they're gonna be here forever and ever.

The end.

Story 2. The girl and the boy were looking through the woods, and they found a alien spaceship.

And a family of aliens came out.

The girl wanted to go pet the dog, but the aliens took her away and brought her into space.

Both of these stories were created by children with specific language impairment, and both show content weaknesses. The first story has a good sense of drama and dialogue, but there is no plot development. The second story conveys a set of connected events occurring over time, but lacks style. The biggest difference between these stories, however, is in grammaticality. The first story has numerous grammatical errors and the second has almost none.

To look more systematically at potential discrepancies between grammaticality and story content, we created an additional scoring option for the self-generated stories in the TNL. Taking items from the TNL score sheet that focused on one or the other of these areas, we created an index that showed the strength of grammaticality relative to content. When we applied this scheme to the Moser (2003) data, a fascinating pattern emerged: children in the SLI group tended to show great disparity between content and grammaticality—in one direction or the other—while the children with normal language development were equally skillful at both aspects of storytelling. Garcia (2005) replicated this study using a somewhat different set of scoring items and found similar patterns of group difference.

When we applied this scheme to the Moser (2003) data, the scores varied from 0 to 86 percent across the 26 children. A clear pattern of difference emerged when we looked at the scores for children from her two groups. Children in the SLI group tended to score either above 60 percent or below 40 percent, indicating that grammaticality was much stronger than content, or vice versa. Children with normal language development, in contrast, tended to have a balanced performance, earning scores between 40 and 60 percent. Garcia (2005) replicated this study using a somewhat different set of scoring items, and found similar, but even stronger, group differences. What is going on here?

The Challenge of Telling a Story

Data from these studies point to group differences in processing capacity. The children with normally developing language apparently had sufficient resources for the narrative task. Some told better stories than others, but at all levels of absolute ability, they handled form and content with equivalent success. The children with SLI presented a different picture. They, too, varied in absolute competence but, regardless of developmental level, the storytelling task seemed to require more resource than was available, forcing them to focus on either content or form. They could concentrate on creating an interesting story and risk grammatical breakdowns, or pay attention to sentence formulation and be satisfied with a more mundane story. (See also Colozzo et al., 2006, for a somewhat different interpretation.)

I am the first to admit that there is much we don't yet understand about the notion of capacity limitations. However, one clear conclusion does emerge from my 20 years of reading on this topic—*capacity* is best defined operationally, as a functional notion. As such, it doesn't necessarily refer to the size of a "bin" or a "pool" that is bigger or smaller, but rather to the amount of work that is doable in a unit of time. Capacity limitations *may* reflect absolute differences in the size of the resource pool, but there are other equally potent explanations. Inefficiency, lack of temporal coordination, slowness, gaps in knowledge, and recall difficulties, to name just a few, could easily limit the amount of work that was doable in a unit of time (i.e., create capacity limitations).

We don't know which of these is the primary problem for children with SLI, or even whether the same explanation will hold for all children in this group. The important point is that from a functional perspective we can view capacity as a consequence rather than a cause. We may be able to increase capacity by changing one of the factors that determines it. Good candidates for our intervention effort are the knowledge schemes that provide the framework for narrative. The normally developing child can acquire these schemes and grammatical patterns simultaneously, but children with SLI have trouble doing so. If we can help children acquire these schemes, we will make narrative processing easier, effectively increasing capacity.

Thinking About Narrative Assessment

Given the inherent complexity of the narrative task, we need to do more than decide whether or not a given child's narratives are age appropriate. We also need to explore the various possible sources of a child's difficulty. Naremore (1997) suggests a series of questions to aid with this task:

- **Could the child have developed the pertinent script?** It would be difficult for me to create a very convincing story about a hunting trip or a dance class, since I know nothing about what goes on in these settings. Maybe we are asking the child to tell or retell a story about an unfamiliar sort of event, thereby removing one important scaffold. We can interview family members or the child to explore this possibility.

- **Can the child indicate knowledge of the script nonverbally?** Even if children have had pertinent experience, they may not have developed a script or be able to employ it when needed. One way to explore this possibility is to create nonverbal activities in which a child can demonstrate script knowledge, such as role playing a trip to the store or arranging sequenced pictures.

- **Can the child convey the script in words?** It may ultimately be the language that is the problem. This can be explored by having the child tape-record an explanation of what happens within a given script, perhaps suggesting that you wish to give it to another child who doesn't know these things. Keep in mind though, that the telling of a script is not yet a story. There is no setting, no problem, no resolution, no art. In this task, the child has only to say what usually happens at, for example, McDonalds, or the movies, or a birthday party.

- **Can the child retell a story based on a known script?** Once we have determined that a child is familiar with a particular script and can recall and put it into words, we can begin to explore his or her knowledge of story forms. The easiest narrative task is one in which the child listens to a story based on the familiar script and then retells it. Again, we need to create a reason for the retelling, perhaps have the child create another tape recording to share with a friend. In any case, the story should consist of one episode with all of its components: setting, problem or initiating event, plan, attempt, outcome, response, and ending. We can note which components of the story are included in the retelling, and listen for language difficulties with reference or cohesion. Keep in mind, however, that this particular version of story grammar is drawn from the Western European cultures and that children from other culture groups may be using a different story scheme.

- **Can the child combine all of this in self-generated narratives?** If we determine that the child has the requisite knowledge bases but still has difficulty telling coherent stories, processing difficulties become the most likely explanation. The best strategy for assessing this possibility is to reduce the processing load and see if the story improves. For example, we could provide external memory supports such as sequenced story pictures (perhaps drawn by the child), rehearse the necessary vocabulary, or play out the script with dolls or action figures just prior to telling the story. We could also discuss various parts of the story with the child in a first telling, then have the child tell the story. If limitations in working memory are at the root of the child's difficulties, these activities should lead to improved narrative performance.

Coda

We generally think of narrative intervention as especially suited for school-age children. But the general frameworks that narratives require (i.e., scripts and story grammars) begin their development during the preschool years. Activities such as role playing and listening to stories—especially those with familiar content, simple sentences, and clear plots—will help preschoolers with language impairments develop these schemes. There are many good sources for story material on the Internet. One site worth a bookmark is www.storynet.org.❖

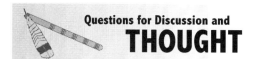

Questions for Discussion and
THOUGHT

1. What narrative tests or other assessment materials are you currently using? Analyze the stories in these materials and rank them for difficulty. Pay attention to (1) number of episodes, (2) availability of visual supports, (3) nature of task (e.g., recall versus creation), and (4) familiarity of the script. Do your materials provide a good range of difficulty or are there gaps?

2. Look at stories produced by children on your caseloads. Do any of them seem to follow the patterns found in Curan et al. (2004), that is, are they strong in content or grammaticality, but not both?

Self-Guided Learning
ACTIVITY

Events can be thought of in very particular or very general ways. We can think about the family trip to Disneyland in 1985, or about trips to amusement parks in general. When we think about amusement parks in a general fashion, we can create a *script* that identifies the nature and order of typical subevents such as: drive to park; stand in line; buy tickets; walk around and investigate; choose a ride; stand in line; go on ride; buy and eat treat; go on more rides; leave park; drive home. In the world of children, other event types that are likely to be the basis of scripts would be going to the doctor, going to a grocery store, going to a restaurant. Think about these general event types and create scripts for each of them.

Issues in Intervention

Early language intervention—the phrase holds such promise and yet there is so much we still do not understand about the process. I returned for my doctorate primarily because I could not explain what I had been doing in the clinic. It was the end of the 1960s. We had studied Chomsky, thought hard about the implications of his theory, and realized we had a problem. If language was indeed hard-wired and language learning was a self-guided process, how could an outside agent have any effect at all? It took me 18 years to answer this question, but I ultimately did, and along the way developed a framework for thinking about early language intervention. The first essay in this section presents this theory. To be productive and creative therapists, able to respond in a unique fashion to each child and each session, we need general principles rather than recipes. "Fit, Focus, and Functionality" is an easy-to-remember formulation of three principles that can and should guide our practice.

The remaining essays in this section address other general aspects of teaching and learning. In Essays 22 and 23, you will discover that I try never to use the word *reinforcement*, and am no fan of Applied Behavior Analysis. Whether or not you come to the same conclusions, you will have a chance to think carefully about children's motivations and about how to evaluate the claims made for therapy programs.

Finally, we come to the holy grail of early intervention—changes in the learning process itself. How wonderful it would be to work ourselves out of a job! This is a challenge we haven't yet solved, but Essay 24 suggests two promising approaches to helping children learn to learn.

21 Fit, Focus, and Functionality: An Essay on Early Language Intervention

NOTE: This essay was first published in 1985 and is reproduced here by permission of the publishers. I have done little updating except for a brief reference to connectionist theories and mention of Leonard's book. There are, of course, many new research findings that could be cited but they would not change the force or general applicability of the framework. I have, however, added a brief addendum to indicate the ways that this intervention theory has evolved since 1985, particularly in regard to older children.

The Nature of Language Learning

Four tenets of contemporary psycholinguistic theory provide the foundation for an intervention model. First, **language is both the product and the tool of intellect.** Language emerges at a predictable stage of intellectual development, when the child has achieved the ability to create symbols, the structural capacity to use tools, the processing skills to analyze complex auditory objects, and an organized treasury of ideas worth talking about. Once language learning begins, the process is guided by cognitive operating principles that are nonverbal in origin (Slobin, 1973; Johnston, 1985a). The language-mind relationships do not just work in one direction, however. Even during the acquisition period, children use their available language skills to represent absent objects and events. It is this representation which makes reflective, analytical thought possible. Children can anticipate the consequences of actions, compare different perspectives or end states, explore new social roles through pretense—all by making use of language symbols. In short, language functions are not insular in nature, but originate from, and interact with, many other aspects of intellect.

Second, **language serves communicative ends and is learned in the course of communication events.** Language may be useful for private reflection, but it is quintessentially social. The system itself is conventional and children learn to speak while interacting with parents, peers, and other members of their social world. Unlike most adult language learners, young children seldom practice language per se. They cannot consider the form of an utterance apart from its message (e.g., deVilliers & deVilliers, 1972) and do not normally attend to utterances spoken without communicative force (Brown, 1973). Instead, young children work out their knowledge of the system while using language to accomplish social purposes such as exchanging information, directing attention, and requesting

155

objects or actions. It is not only that the desire to communicate provides a necessary impetus for language learning. Certain grammatical patterns can be discovered only in the context of communication because they are functional in nature (Bates & MacWhinney, 1982).

Third, **language learning is an active, abstracting process.** Whether we characterize the learning as rule formulation or as an emergence of connectionist networks, it requires selectivity and prioritization, and yields representations that are necessarily abstract. Competent language users must know the abstract combinatorial patterns and form-classes that comprise the structure of a language, otherwise they could not process the infinite number of novel utterances that human communication requires. Children, of course, never meet these abstract categories directly. No red light identifies words that are nouns; no single physical form marks the subject of a sentence. Word classes such as noun, grammatical categories such as subject, order rules, and so forth must be created as the young learner notes organizational similarities across utterances (Brown, 1973; MacWhinney, 1982). This sort of learning exceeds the power of traditional stimulus-response accounts and demands that we view the learner as ultimately responsible for his or her own growth.

Lastly, **language acquisition is a self-regulated process.** This principle has been implicit in the preceding three, but it deserves further attention. If children express only the meanings they understand, if children learn language to accomplish their own social purposes, if children construct abstract categories, then we should not be surprised to find that they select their own learning goals and proceed at their own pace. Language development provides an excellent example of what cognitivists call top-down processing (Norman, 1976). At every point children use what they already know about the world and about language to analyze new linguistic data. When the necessary interpretive tools are lacking, children fail to comprehend a speech event and there is little impact on knowledge. On the other hand, when prerequisite interpretive knowledge routines are available, children begin to notice, analyze, and organize new sorts of linguistic phenomena. Instances of such selectivity abound throughout the child language literature. Note, for example, children's relatively late acquisition of the English auxiliary DO. This word in its main verb, agentive sense is an early achievement. Despite lexical availability, however, auxiliary functions for DO are not learned until after children have acquired other members of the auxiliary verb class which have clearer functions and less complex syntactic properties (Brown, 1973). Children's acquisition of language is predictable and systematic exactly because their available knowledge at any point largely determines what they are capable of learning next.

These four tenets of modern language acquisition theory have far-reaching implications for the instructional goals and methods of a language intervention program. Before considering these implications, however, we need to establish the character of developmental language disorders. Does the view of language learning discussed above pertain to children with specific learning disabilities in the area of language?

The Nature of Language Disorders

Broadly defined, the purpose of any developmental intervention is to accelerate or to redirect the course of learning. In the case of children with language impairment, research to date indicates that language learning is late and slow but not off-course, so only the first intervention goal pertains. Language-impaired children violate none of the tenets of child language theory discussed above. They exhibit the same sort of relationships between thought and language, use language for a variety of social purposes, show normal sequences in the order of acquisition for specific language forms within domain, and generate novel utterances that reveal their knowledge of abstract patterns (see Leonard, 1998 for a review). This is not to say that their language learning is ordinary. Children with language impairment are remarkably slow in their discovery of language patterns. The key symptom of language disorder is thus a developmental gap between language knowledge and achievement in other areas of learning (i.e., conceptual, social, motor-perceptual). The source of language learning difficulties is as yet unknown, although the most compelling explanations currently center on information processing deficits.

The challenge of language intervention is to simplify the learning task without changing its basic character. If the child is to achieve linguistic competence, language learning must remain integrated with intellect, motivated by communication, actively inductive, and self-directed. But if we are to achieve true intervention, language learning must also be facilitated in specific, well-calculated ways. The challenge for educators is to manage this tension between the common and the extraordinary. What sort of intervention program can maintain the essence of language learning and yet accelerate it?

The Nature of Preschool Language Intervention

Three concepts provide the keys to successful language intervention with the preschool-age child: *fit, focus, and functionality.* I have argued earlier that language learning is energized by the child's own social needs, utilizes his own cognitive resources, and is guided by his own search for the means to express particular ideas. This self-regulation implies that **instructional goals in language intervention must fit the child's social purposes, interpretive resources, and emergent meanings.** When instructional experiences are designed to advance the child's knowledge one step beyond its current level, learning is more likely to occur (Kuhn, 1972; Johnston, 1982b). When new information is pertinent to the child's plan of the moment, attentional resources are conserved (Hoff-Ginsberg & Shatz, 1982).

Children acquire grammatical patterns in a generally predictable sequence; this fact might suggest the grouping of pupils by language level. Prior linguistic knowledge is, however, just one determinant of a child's readiness to learn a given language pattern. We must also consider nonverbal knowledge and communicative intentions. These parameters combine in so many ways as to virtually preclude a common set of intervention goals. We can maximize the speed of language learning by designing thoroughly individualized instructional programs.

The content of language intervention is not the only area where appropriateness is crucial. Self-regulation also implies that instructional methods in language intervention must fit the child's cognitive style. Two aspects of early cognition impinge on our method. First, it seems that individual children approach the language object with different processing strategies. They may, for instance, acquire large sentence-like units which they then disassemble, or they may acquire word-like units from which they build up longer strings (Peters, 1973). They may assume that language serves primarily expressive, social functions, or they may assume that its primary utility is descriptive and referential (Nelson, 1973). Second, preschool language learning appears to be largely incidental in nature. As noted earlier, children acquire language while communicating. Formal properties of the system are secondary to messages, and there are few signs that the young child thinks much about talking. This may be due to the fact that language is by definition a symbolic tool, a means to some other end. If children were to focus exclusively on the shape of the tool, its symbolic function might be lost. Alternatively, the incidental nature of language learning may reflect the metacognitive limitations of early childhood. Young children may be unable to step aside and consider the way an idea could be expressed apart from the actual act of expression. In either case, the incidental character of early language learning springs directly from essential qualities of language and of the learner.

The instructional costs of ignoring these two aspects of cognitive style could be great. Nelson (1973), for example, argues from her longitudinal data that early language learning is more rapid when maternal language use is consonant with the child's strategies. And at least one study has demonstrated that language rules are learned more quickly when used communicatively than when explicitly practiced (Murray, 1972, as cited in Ruder and Smith, 1974). Even though we have much to learn about cognitive style, it seems more likely that we will maximize the speed of language learning if we recognize differences in strategies and work within the constraints of incidental learning.

Instructional methods in language intervention not only must fit the learner's cognitive style, they must compensate for information-processing deficits. Here the notion of focus comes into play. Current theorists agree that language learning is essentially an organizing and abstracting process. The human mind is predisposed to search out the regular patterns which underlie the utterances that children hear. Abstract categories of forms emerge according to relative position, meaning, or other characteristics. Ordinarily this search for regularity must be conducted across utterances of great diversity, and over large expanses of time. **Language intervention must therefore utilize focused linguistic input, to narrow the child's search for order and simplify the organizing task.**

The selection of an instructional goal initiates focus; the construction of the language learning event embodies it. By manipulating the frequency, salience, and context of forms, the interventionist can draw the child's attention to pertinent data. Teachers can, for instance, present many examples of a targeted language pattern without interspersing other sorts of utterances. This strategy facilitates internal comparisons and allows for economical mental sets (Bock, 1982). Teachers can also present targeted forms in sentence-final or stressed positions. Even the copula can be thus presented with some discourse creativity. Imagine a playful argument in which the teacher responds to the child's "He's big" with "He *is?*" or "He *is* big." Given our natural processing disposition towards novelty and recency, such discourse manipulations attract the mind's eye to critical language facts (Norman, 1976). Finally, teachers can present their linguistic models in the context of events which make the meaning transparent (i.e., events which are interpretable, invite a particular perspective, and lie within the child's attentional flow). This strategy simplifies the child's first-priority language task of finding meaning, and thereby frees the mental resources needed for a rapid analysis of the fading acoustic event (Hoff-Ginsberg & Shatz, 1982).

Techniques of this sort have had demonstrable accelerating effects on language learning in normal children (e.g., Hoff-Ginsberg & Shatz, 1982; Leonard, 1975; Nelson, 1976; Newport et al., 1977). They well serve the needs of language-disordered children who suffer apparent processing deficits. By increasing the concentration and salience of a particular utterance type in contexts which clarify meaning, we can (1) reduce demands on attention and memory, (2) provide both positional and semantic cues to structure, and thus (3) maximize the likelihood that the targeted pattern will be learned.

Such linguistic engineering may be preplanned. The interventionist can select an instructional goal based upon the child's prior achievements and contrive a communication game which demands use of the targeted pattern. The real strength of this approach to intervention, however, is that it can also be used in completely natural child-initiated activities. Interventionists need not always take children away from their practical and social activities; they can bring the language lesson to the world of the young child.

What is this child's world? In our culture it is largely the world of play, where activities are chosen by the player and pursued for their intrinsic value. These play activities are, of course, the occasion for intellectual and social-affective growth. Young children learn about relationships and classes while pursuing such practical and mundane tasks as building block towers or baking cookies. They explore social roles through pretend play or through the negotiations inherent in cooperative ventures. It is exactly in this world of practical and social purposes that children learn to speak. Their need to explain, to understand, to direct, to request, to hold in mind, to imagine, or to transform keeps them grappling with the language object. Language has a functional character. We do things with words. This being true, **language intervention must provide children with functional language tools.**

A survey of current intervention practice suggests two ways in which this might be accomplished (Weber-Olson & Ruder, 1984). The interventionist could estimate the child's communicative needs and teach forms which are *likely* to be functional. Alternatively, the interventionist could accompany children as they pursue their practical goals and provide examples of just those language forms which the children *do in fact* need. The second approach more fully exploits the motive force of verbal instrumentality. Likewise, the interventionist could have children practice language forms and then incorporate them back into communication. Or, the interventionist could, from the start, work through activities that require genuine, communicative use of language. Again, the second approach more fully exploits the functionality of language.

Messages can be considered in the abstract, but as such they have little compelling power. It is my belief that children will learn language more readily when they see it function in the moment, when specific utterances spring directly from specific communicative intents, and when these intents are drawn from the world of the child. This latter point is particularly crucial for language-disordered children whose communicative intents may far exceed their expressive abilities. Their educational milieu must provide opportunities for advanced level practical actions while accepting and modeling rather primitive utterances.

Summary and Conclusions

This essay has attempted to characterize an approach to language intervention which seems particularly well suited to the needs of preschool-age children with language disorders. It reflects both what we know to be true of language learning and what we know of these children. This view of early language intervention can be summarized by the following set of operating principles (in the style of Slobin, 1973):

(A) **Operating Principles in regard to Content Fit**

   1. Teach language that expresses the child's available meanings.

   2. Teach language that accomplishes the child's desired purposes.

   3. Teach language that the child can interpret given his or her current knowledge of language and of the world.

(B) **Operating Principles in regard to Style Fit**

   4. Teach language recognizing the child's preferred strategies.

   5. Teach language while seeming to pursue some other goal.

(C) **Operating Principles in regard to Focus**

    6. Teach language by providing concentrated, salient examples of a single pattern.

    7. Teach language in contexts which clarify meaning.

(D) **Operating Principles in regard to Functionality**

    8. Teach language in natural as well as contrived transactions.

    9. Teach language while communicating real messages.

    10. Teach language in the child's world.

What does it mean to *teach* when only the child can construct the abstract patterns which ensure creative language use? And what does such teaching look like? Given the view of language learning discussed here, a language interventionist teaches by creating physical, communicative, and linguistic environments in which the child can easily learn. These occasions for learning will be infinitely diverse in surface form; they may involve any number of people in the child's world, occur any place the child travels, emerge out of any sphere of activity. Language intervention is best understood, not as a set of lesson plans or program descriptions, but as a set of principles which apply for all language-disordered children, in all settings. My goal in this essay has been to develop one such—admittedly naïve—theory of language intervention, arguing both from prior theoretical commitments and from empirical findings. It is my belief that such efforts bring coherence and creativity to our instructional practice.

Addendum

It has now been some 20 years since this essay was written and I have had much opportunity to discuss the theory with clinical colleagues and see it in action. If I were to rewrite the essay today, the substantive changes would be elaborations, not revisions. First, I would expand the section on focus to include more ideas on how it is possible to simplify the learning task through discourse engineering. For example, we now have a better understanding of the ways that linguistic context and content familiarity can influence the earliest uses of a new language form. The literature on processing tradeoffs suggests that we should use familiar words when introducing new sentence patterns, and that we should simplify syntax when introducing new words. You will find this facilitation strategy, and many others, discussed throughout this book. Second, I would extend the theory to include school-age children, with their new resources and new challenges. With older children, my approach would remain primarily communication centered, but there would now be opportunity for the occasional explicit talk about talking. The only major additions to the theory would concern mastery learning, and the need to target improved language performance, as well as the learning of new forms. With preschool-age children, we primarily focus on the initial acquisition of language forms; with school-age children, we also need to focus on the child's control of, and access to, this knowledge. Again, you will find ideas about the later stages of learning in many of the essays in this book.❖

From "Fit, Focus, and Functionality: An Essay on Early Language Intervention," by J. Johnston, 1985b, *Child Language Teaching and Therapy, 1*(2), pp. 125–134. © 1985 by Child Language Teaching and Therapy. Reprinted with permission.

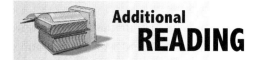

Additional
READING

Ellis Weismer, S. (1990-1991). Theory and practice: A principled approach to treatment of young children with specific language disorders. *National Student Speech Language Hearing Association Journal, 18,* 76–86.

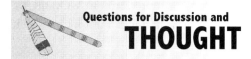

Questions for Discussion and
THOUGHT

1. The opening sections of the essay mention some of the early intellectual and social tasks that are made possible by language. Review these tasks and think about the experiences of young children who do not have language. What sorts of social and cognitive limitations would they face?

2. The essay mentions acquisition of DO as evidence in support of self-regulation. Can you think of other language acquisition facts that seem to reflect the child's own agenda?

3. Take turns describing recent therapy sessions. Identify elements of the sessions that were ordinary/common and those that were extraordinary/therapeutic.

4. The essay illustrates how we can manipulate word position and stress to create facilitative discourse. What other aspects of language can we manipulate to make it easier to learn?

5. The essay argues that therapy needs to involve the communicative use of language, but doesn't need to be naturalistic. Would this be equally true at all ages?

6. The fit, focus, and functionality (FFF) operating principles apply to all children regardless of diagnosis. Does that mean the SLP does the same thing with each child?

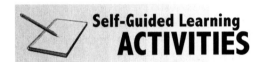

Self-Guided Learning
ACTIVITIES

1. Observe a colleague or student conduct a language learning task (or session). Evaluate the task using the FFF framework. Is it in accord with the operating principles at the end of article? If not, think about what its general principles might be. If the SLP wanted to change the activity so that it was more in accord with FFF, what might she or he do?

2. Write a one-paragraph summary of the FFF operating principles that could be given to special educators and other professionals. If you are hesitant about FFF, write a paragraph about an approach you are more familiar with, taking this essay as an example. What are the assumptions and general principles that determine the approach?

22 Reinforcement or Motivation?

I once banned the word *reinforcement* from my classroom. I wanted students to find a synonym for this word and in the process reflect on its meaning. Which would you choose as a synonym: *extrinsic reward* or *motivation?* Our preferences for one or the other of these words indicate something important about our views of learning. The words *extrinsic reward* and *reinforcement* refer to things that are external to the child, and are controlled by people in the child's social environment. Educators who are committed to these concepts believe that teachers, SLPs, and parents can somehow ensure that learning occurs. The word *motivation,* on the other hand, refers to the child's *own* reasons for learning. Motivation is not something controlled from the outside. We may look for what motivates a child and use that information to create attractive learning tasks, but it is the *child's* interests and values that ultimately fuel the learning. Given that language development is self-regulated and that language representations are necessarily abstract, the notion of *motivation* seems more harmonious with the process of language learning than does the notion of *reinforcement.* We may provide lessons for the child with language deficiencies but ultimately it is the child who must decide—and work—to learn.

Why then does the term *reinforcement* continue in widespread use among SLPs? One reason is that the notion of reinforcement, particularly in educational settings, has lost much of its theoretical grounding. Most SLPs would side with Chomsky in his critical rejection of Skinner's view of language development. Many of them nevertheless favor the use of extrinsic reward systems such as stickers or game boards and believe that these items "reinforce" children's learning. If you ask an SLP why she talks about *reinforcement,* she might explain that children with learning difficulties need extra support. If you ask further whether she believes that behavioral change *will* always occur as a direct function of the reinforcement, she is likely to say no. Skinner might be surprised at this response, but for many educators, the word *reinforcement* means *encouragement* and nothing more.

If extrinsic reward systems were benign, the story might end here. We could merely smile at the way that the language of behaviorism has outlived the theory, and buy more stickers. However, a long line of research studies cautions us to be more thoughtful about this decision.

Undermining Intrinsic Motivation

Lepper, Greene, and Nisbett (1973) were the first to explore the effects of extrinsic reward systems on preschoolers. After observing the spontaneous play patterns of children in a nursery school, these researchers identified 55 children who showed strong preferences for drawing activities during periods of free play. They then assigned these children to one of three groups, matching the groups for gender, age, classroom, and the length of the initial observation period. One group of children was invited to accompany the experimenter into a special playroom and was told that each child would be given a prize for drawing pictures. They drew the pictures and received the prize. A second group of children also went to the playroom, drew pictures, and received a prize, but these children did not know about the reward until after their drawings were completed. The third group of children went to the playroom with the experimenter and drew pictures, but received no prize.

Two weeks later, the children were observed in their classrooms by research assistants who were blind to group membership. The startling result was that the children who had drawn the pictures knowing that they would receive a reward were now drawing less frequently than they had done prior to the experiment. Similar declines were not seen for children in the other two groups. Needless to say, this study caused a sensation. How could extrinsic rewards (i.e., reinforcement) *lessen* the likelihood of a behavior? Lepper et al. (1973) argued that the rewards had changed the children's perception of drawing activities. Instead of being intrinsically interesting, drawing had become merely the instrumental means to a reward.

Was Lepper, Greene, and Nisbett a Fluke?

I recently discovered a meta-analysis (Deci et al., 1999) of experiments on the effects of extrinsic reward systems since Lepper et al. (1973). The authors reviewed 128 studies spanning 16 years! The results of this long line of investigation are fascinating. The authors summarize their findings as follows:

> In general, tangible rewards had a significant *negative* effect on intrinsic motivation for interesting tasks, and this effect showed up with participants ranging from preschool to college, with interesting activities ranging from word games to construction puzzles, and with various rewards ranging from dollar bills to marshmallows. (p. 653)

The researchers conducted a number of subanalyses to look at different types of rewards, different contingencies, and different groups of participants. The results of these comparisons add depth to the overall summary. First, participants responded differently to tangible rewards versus verbal rewards, and to expected rewards versus unexpected rewards. Tangible rewards, when they were announced prior to the activity and thus were expected, consistently undermined intrinsic motivation. Positive verbal feedback, on the other hand, seemed to enhance motivation, at least for college students. The authors suggest, however, that this finding may only reflect the fact that verbal praise usually cannot be expected. This interpretation was confirmed in the three studies where participants were told ahead of time that they would receive verbal feedback. These studies again reported a reduction in motivation.

Some of the most interesting findings for early interventionists concern age differences. Deci and his colleagues found that, overall, children were much more likely than college students to experience the detrimental effects of tangible rewards and to show a significant decrease in activities they had once preferred. Moreover, these effects showed up in posttests that occurred two weeks after the rewards had been given, indicating that the changes in behavior could not be attributed to some transitory state such as satiation. The meta-analysis also found that children never show the enhancing effect of verbal rewards, perhaps because children are less able to separate the informational aspects of verbal feedback from its controlling aspects.

Finally, the researchers looked at reward contingencies by grouping studies according to whether rewards were given for mere participation, for task completion, or for some standard of performance. The results here are quite sobering for us as educators.

> By far the most detrimental type of performance-contingent reward, indeed the most detrimental type of reward, is one that is commonly used in applied settings, namely one in which rewards are administered as a direct function of people's performance. If people do superlatively, they get large rewards, but if they do not display optimal performance, they get smaller rewards. (Deci et al., 1999, p. 644)

The Big Picture

Many educators will find this body of research disturbing. To be sure, the experiments have only considered interesting tasks. But there is no comfort in the few studies that have looked at the effects of rewards on tasks that were not interesting. They find that while intrinsic motivation for interesting tasks is undermined by tangible rewards, boring tasks are not affected one way or the other—they merely remain boring.

To return to my opening thoughts, what is at issue here is ultimately our views on the nature of teaching and learning. Or, as Deci and colleagues (1999) frame it, the rewards debate is really a debate about "the control versus self-determination of human behavior in social contexts" (p. 658). It is easy to get caught up in our perceptions of deficit and difficulty, and forget that virtually all children find pleasure in competence and want to learn. In my 17 years of clinical practice, I can think of only one child who might challenge that claim, and even then I must admit that my interventions may have been part of the problem. Our role as teachers and facilitators is to make learning possible, to offer tasks that make sense and fit the child's competencies, to lead the child to new places and ideas one step at a time. In the process we may need to give up our desire to take credit for progress, forget reinforcement, and be content to merely watch as children learn.

Understanding the child's interests and capabilities requires ingenuity and insight. One of my favorite examples of clinical imagination concerns a 10-year-old child I will call Tony, who lived in a rural midsized town. In today's scheme, Tony would fall on the autistic spectrum, with low-normal IQ scores and language learning difficulties. What made Tony exceptional was his passion for buses. He was so focused on buses that he knew the personal history of every bus in town—which seats had been repaired, which windows had been replaced, old numbering schemes—you name it, Tony knew it. He talked incessantly about the buses, and to some clinicians this would have been a problem. His SLP, however, chose to view this knowledge as an asset. Tony's learning goal was question patterns, so together with his clinician he prepared and rehearsed a question-filled interview for the one person in town who knew more about the buses than Tony did—the maintenance supervisor at the bus barn. I wish I could have sat in the corner and listened when these two bus fanatics met. I do know that Tony needed no extrinsic rewards for this activity.

So what shall it be? Reinforcement or motivation? I know that we cannot change the whole educational establishment and the many ways in which it undermines the intrinsic motivation that young children bring to the classroom. But for me, 128 studies pointing in the same direction make a persuasive case. At the very least they argue for caution in the use of extrinsic rewards, and clear vision as we look for each child's path to learning.❖

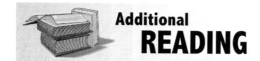

Additional
READING

White, R. W. (1959). Motivation reconsidered: The concept of competence. *Psychological Review, 66,* 297–333

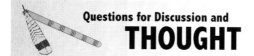

Questions for Discussion and
THOUGHT

1. Many children on the autism spectrum get stuck on particular activities or ideas. When should we ignore these obsessions? Try to extinguish them? Use them as motivators?

2. What aspects of the typical primary classroom seem most likely to dampen a child's natural pleasure in learning?

3. Given the research summarized here, extrinsic reward systems seem to have a large cost. Do they also have a benefit? Do the benefits ever outweigh the costs (i.e., are there circumstances that warrant extrinsic rewards)?

Identify the child on your caseload that seems to have the least motivation to learn.

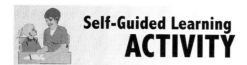

Self-Guided Learning
ACTIVITY

Make every effort to find out what that child's primary interests are. Ask the child, child's friends, family, or teacher what the child *really* likes. Now, plan and carry out a lesson that incorporates these interests in every possible way. Do you see any changes in the child's involvement in the learning tasks?

23 ABA Revisited

Autism is on our minds these days. Due to broadened criteria and public awareness, the number of children receiving this diagnosis has increased dramatically. While there seems to be a consensus about the need for early and intensive intervention, there is no consensus about the nature of the programs. The range of options is staggering—from highly structured applied-behaviorism to play therapy, from home to center, from professional to volunteer worker.

My introduction to autism was with a three-year-old named Etta. It was 1968 and Lovaas had just published the results from his behavior modification treatments of autism (Lovaas et al., 1966). My clinic hired one of his doctoral students as a consultant and began to provide speech-language therapy for young children with autism according to the Lovaas model. Etta's program included both individual sessions and nursery school activities, for a total of 14 to 17 hours a week. I was Etta's SLP, and for more than a year, she and I did battle over breakfast and a range of learning tasks. I demanded and she resisted. As far as I could see, she made no progress in our program, speaking only once during the entire period, "Mommy. Go home." With hindsight, I could say that Etta's global delay accounted for her lack of progress. But more honestly, I must say that we knew nothing about the early cognitive and social accomplishments that prepare the way for language, and were not yet thinking developmentally about young children with autism. The result was a program that did not fit Etta's needs.

My experience with Etta has been echoed by many of my students who have volunteered as therapists in Applied Behavioral Analysis (ABA) programs, the current incarnation of the Lovaas approach. A substantial number, though not all, tell stories like my story of Etta. It is now, however, no longer 1968. We can draw on nearly four decades of research about early development and the communication and learning patterns of children with autism. Increasingly, this knowledge is being translated into programs and outcome research. It is time to revisit ABA.

ABA

Like all therapy programs, Applied Behavioral Analysis entails a set of procedures and content features that are bundled together—but needn't be. Traditional ABA programs are highly structured, teacher-directed, decontextualized, and developmentally uninformed. They also present behavioral tasks one at a time, use extrinsic rewards, and repeat a given task until the child reaches a specific level of performance. It is easy to imagine a program that would have some, but not all of these features, for example, one that is highly structured but does not use extrinsic rewards, or one that presents discrete learning trials but orders them according to developmental norms. There is by now a large body of reports that document the efficacy of the ABA approach for many children with autism. However, most of these outcome studies are not designed to pinpoint the specific features of the program that are responsible for its success—and it is virtually certain that the various features are not equally potent. I think it is important that we consider alternate versions of a program whenever research suggests ways to improve them. I am going to talk about some features of the traditional ABA model that I believe should be changed. For readers who, like myself, are not behaviorists, the features I will be discussing could be incorporated into other programs as well.

First Things First

One good candidate for change in the ABA model is the focus on speech itself. SLPs and other language specialists are often called to work with children with autism who are not yet speaking. For such children, traditional ABA programs begin immediate work on speech sounds and words, but the developmental literature indicates that aspects of nonverbal communication would make better learning goals. Well before their first birthday, normally developing children establish and maintain joint attention. They show off, follow the gaze patterns of others, hold up objects for mutual appreciation, point, and ultimately engage in the shifting eye patterns that mean "Hey, do you see this?" or "How about some help with the juice?" These moments of shared attention are not only excellent opportunities for language learning, they are evidence of the child's emergent understanding of like mind and common experience. Such understanding is central to social relationships and provides many of our reasons to talk.

A substantial number of studies now show that the preverbal ability to create and sustain joint attention is one of the best predictors of language development in children with autism. One of the most recent was conducted by a British team (Charman et al., 2003) who identified a group of children with autism/PDD at 20 months of age, and assessed their ability in the areas of joint attention, play, imitation, and IQ. The children were assessed again at 42 months to determine the links between these variables and later language growth. Joint attention was measured by having a series of large mechanical toys move around the room and observing the child to see if he or she shifted eye gaze from the toy to the adult and back. Imitation was measured by modeling an action with a novel object three times and seeing whether the child would repeat it. The researchers found that performance on both of these measures predicted receptive language abilities at 42 months. It has not been shown yet that language learning in nonverbal children with autism can be accelerated by fostering joint attention, but it seems like a good bet.

Who Decides?

A second feature of ABA programs that we might wish to change is the directive character of the interactions. Our cues here come from a recent study of the role of parents in facilitating episodes of joint attention. Observations of normally developing children had shown that even before an infant learns to follow the gaze of others or alternate gaze between caretaker and object, mothers create moments of shared attention by focusing on whatever has already engaged the child's interest. Siller and Sigman (2002) wondered whether caretakers of children with autism would do likewise, especially given their child's delays in this area. The research team video-taped three groups of children as they interacted with their caretakers: 25 children with autism, 18 children with developmental delays, and 18 children with normal development, all at an MA of 24 months. The taped interactions were then analyzed to determine the degree to which caretakers pointed to, showed, offered, or talked about toys to which the child was already attending. All children in the study were also assessed for language and cognitive levels, and the children with autism were reevaluated 1, 10, and 16 years later.

Two important findings emerged from these data. First, the caregivers of children with autism synchronized their behavior to their children's attention patterns just as much as did caretakers of children in the other two groups. There was no indication here that caregivers were responsible for their children's social and cognitive delays. Second, caretakers who showed higher degrees of synchronization at the 24-month session, had children who had made greater gains in initiating joint attention 1 year later. Moreover, caregivers who showed more *verbal* synchronization at 24 months had children who made greater gains in language over 10 and 16 years. This was particularly true if the caretakers' comments allowed the child to maintain rather than switch their focus of attention. Moments of joint attention that preserve the child's prior focus may require fewer cognitive resources and/or allow the child's own interests to motivate learning. Either of these mechanisms would increase the likelihood of language being learned. We can't prove such causal chains with correlational data, but the strength of the observed linkage is impressive.

This idea of following the child's lead has even been embraced by some educators within the behavioral tradition. Delprato (2001) contrasts the traditional discrete-trial (ABA) approach with what he calls "normalized behavioral intervention." Although still relying on extrinsic rewards and targeting behavioral change, therapists in this second approach work within the child's natural environment and select learning-goals-of-the-moment according to the child's interests and focus of attention. Delprato summarizes 10 studies that directly compared the two types of speech-language therapy. In 8 of the studies, the normalized program produced better language performance and/or generalization, and led to a greater reduction in problem behavior. The remaining 2 studies looked at parental stress instead of the children's language. Here again, parents in the normalized program evidenced less stress, more interest, and greater satisfaction in interacting with their children than parents participating in a more traditional discrete-trial program. Many of these studies involve only a few cases but the research is well designed and the consistency of the findings is ultimately convincing.

Supporting the Emergence of Joint Attention

The research summarized above, along with many more studies cited in each of these articles, suggests that nonverbal children with autism would benefit from therapy that differs from traditional ABA methods: (1) in targeting the domain of joint attention rather than speech itself, (2) in being responsive rather than directive, and (3) in providing caregiver training in natural environments. Two recent reports of therapy outcomes confirm the merit of these ideas.

Whalen and Schreibman (2003) describe a behavior modification program (of the normalized, child-directed type) designed to train joint attention. Three of the four children who completed the program showed generalized gains in joint attention *responses* that were still present three months following treatment. Gains in joint attention *initiations* were more modest, but also present. Interestingly, in posttest ratings by naive observers, all of the participants were rated as improved, and two of the four were judged to be similar to normally developing children matched for LA and MA at about 15 months of age. Here is a summary of program steps:

1. **Responding to joint attention bids** of the trainer—child is expected to look at new toy with increasingly demanding prompts, as follows:

   a. While child is playing with one toy, adult puts child's hand on a different toy as an invitation to switch attention.

   b. As above, but adult merely taps on new toy.

   c. As above, but adult shows new toy to child.

   d. While child is playing with toy, adult requests eye contact, then turns head and points to another object in room.

   e. As above, but adult only uses gaze with no pointing.

2. **Initiating joint attention** based on normal data—child is expected to bid within 10 seconds of beginning play with a toy, using one of the following behaviors:

   - Coordinated gaze shift—object to adult to object (trained with physical and verbal prompts)

   - Pointing at something to capture adult attention (trained with physical and verbal prompts)

This program is still too unmotivated for me, but it does incorporate developmental research into the behavior paradigm, is play based, and allows the child some choices in activity. Whalen and Schreibman (2003) comment that their program would have been improved with a parent training component, and indeed this feature is the centerpiece of a second recent study.

Drew et al. (2002) designed a "social-pragmatic joint attention focused" program in which SLPs visited homes for a three hour session every six weeks for a year. They advised, demonstrated activities, and collaborated with the parent in setting goals for the coming month. Families were encouraged to spend 30 to 60 minutes a day in dedicated teaching time, as well as to act on teachable moments throughout the day. Language gains after one year were greater in the group receiving the social-pragmatic parent training in comparison to a group that had no social-pragmatic parent training but did have equivalent amounts of speech-language therapy, preschool classes, and parental teaching. Drew et al. describe the content of their program as follows:

- Advice about behavioral management

- Explicit teaching of joint attention behaviors such as index finger pointing, gaze switching, showing/holding out objects to adults (Activities included mirror games, pointing to request names while reading picture books, saying, "look" and pointing to things the child likes, and gaze switching games with bubbles.)

- Visual supports for spoken language

- Teaching of enactive and representational gestures through songs, rhymes, and social routines

- Emphasis on nonverbal requests, object function play, imitating actions, and turn taking games

- Wholistic language learning supported through exaggerated prosody

- Analytic language learning supported through repetitive paraphrasing

Lessons Learned

We have much to learn about helping children with autism find their way into the social world. Still, when I look at modern autism research and reflect on my year with Etta, I see that we have been moving in the right direction. Most of us now view speech as inherently communicative. We recognize the larger social and developmental contexts in which language emerges, and we have considerable knowledge of the child and environmental variables that interact in language learning. Each content feature of the Drew et al. (2002) program reflects a substantial body of developmental research with both typical and atypical children. Most of us would now agree with a recent report from National Research Council which concluded that "early intervention is viewed most appropriately as an individualized strategy...based on the science of early childhood development" (Shonkoff & Phillips, 2000, p. 32). I now know what that means. I wish I had learned it sooner.❖

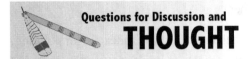

Questions for Discussion and
THOUGHT

1. Select another broad approach to language intervention that you are familiar with (e.g., milieu therapy, Hanen program). What are the bundled features of this approach? Is it child-centered or adult-centered? Does it use language communicatively or not? Does it require the child to talk? What sort of motivation does it rely on? Once you have listed the bundled features of the program, try changing them—one at a time.

2. This essay describes a change in my understanding of the therapeutic process. Look back over the last decade and identify the most important thing you have learned as a result of working as an SLP. After each member of the group shares an answer to this question, reflect on the set of answers. How are answers the same, or different? Are these things that could only be learned on the job, by an experienced SLP, by an older person?

3. What is your experience, and advice, concerning collaborations with someone (e.g., teacher, parent, OT) who holds theoretical views that conflict with your views?

Self-Guided Learning
ACTIVITY

Make a videotape of yourself interacting with a young child either (1) in a play-based therapy session with a preschooler, or (2) in an unstructured conversation with a school-age child. For the first half of the tape, try to synchronize your activity to the child's activity (i.e., follow the child's lead either verbally or nonverbally). For the second half of the tape, stop trying to follow the child's lead and take more initiative. View the tape. Does the child's behavior change from the first to the second part of the session?

24 Do Toddlers Learn to Learn?

During my years at Indiana University, I had many long conversations with Linda Smith, a developmental psychologist who was particularly interested in lexical development. As we explored the relationships between words and ideas, I was always impressed with her ability to turn theoretical possibilities into experimental tasks that even a two-year-old could understand. Linda has recently reported three studies of lexical learning that are elegant, convincing, and directly applicable to our practice. Let me tell you about them.

The Debate

The three studies address a core issue in child language theory, namely, the origins of the toddler's remarkable ability to learn new words. The facts are not in dispute: at a very early age, children exhibit learning strategies that are domain-specific. If you show them a new *u*-shaped, wooden object and say, "This is a dax," they will immediately choose other *u*-shaped objects as further instances of dax, regardless of size or material. This shape bias is, however, only seen in the domain of naming. If you show children the same set of objects, but say only, "Look at this. Get me one," they will *not* preferentially select objects that are the same shape. There seems to be a specific strategy for learning new words that leads children to pay attention to object shape. This bias will not help them learn every sort of word, but for common nouns that refer to concrete objects—the core of a two-year-old's vocabulary—it works very well.

Child language theorists explain the existence of these smart strategies in two very different ways. One group argues that such sophisticated learning in a toddler could only be the result of neural prewiring. The other group argues that infants do not need to come equipped with the strategy itself because general cognitive processes can give rise to specific strategies through experience. This is obviously a key debate and one that has important implications for intervention. If impaired word learning reflects the absence of innately provided strategies, our therapeutic options would seem to be quite limited. If, on the other hand, these language learning strategies are themselves learned, they would seem to be important targets for intervention.

Thinking About Child Language

The Experiments

As one of the theorists in the second group, Linda Smith became convinced that the same-shape bias was actually a byproduct of the child's earliest word learning experiences. Many first words refer to categories of rigid objects that are similar in shape. As children go about the business of figuring out the meanings of these first object labels, they repeatedly hear phrases such as "This is a _____" or "Look. Here's a _____." They also discover from new word to new word that shape is a highly useful cue to the reference object class. Perhaps the phrases used for naming become linked to the notion of shape through general associative learning processes while children are learning their very first words.

To investigate this possibility, Linda and her colleagues (2001) decided to try to find the point at which children first begin to use the same-shape strategy in naming. They observed eight children longitudinally from 15 to 20 months of age. Every three weeks the children would come into the lab and participate in a novel word-learning task. The experimenter would hold up an object saying, for example, "This is a dax." Then, while still holding up the model, she would put out her other hand and say, "Give me a dax. Give me another dax." The children would then select an object from an array of three objects, one of which was like the dax in shape, and two of which resembled the model in some feature other than shape. Throughout the 5-month period, the parents also kept a record of all new words spoken by their child. At the beginning of the study, none of the children knew more than 15 words; by the end of the study each of them knew at least 150 words. Similarly, at 15 months there was no evidence of a same-shape strategy; but by 20 months the children were clearly selecting referents according to shape more often than according to color or texture. Most importantly, when these two areas of learning were compared over time, it turned out that children only started choosing objects by same shape *after* they knew 50 count nouns.

To confirm these longitudinal findings, Linda and her colleagues then conducted a cross-sectional study with 64 children ages 18 to 25 months. They wanted to be sure that their first results were not the product of repeated lab visits, and also to be sure that the early biases they had observed were indeed specific to language learning. In this second study, all of the children's parents completed the vocabulary inventory from the CDI and all of the children participated in the "Give me ___" task. Half of the children participated in the standard, naming version of the task and the other half in a neutral, nonnaming version. Again the results were clear. The same-shape strategy for learning new words was seen only in the children who knew at least 50 count nouns, and it indeed occurred only in the context of naming.

Now comes the really interesting part. In order to move beyond mere correlation, the Indiana researchers conducted a training study. That is to say, they intervened. Ten toddlers, age 17 months, came to the lab weekly for seven weeks. In individual play sessions they were introduced to four novel object categories with their associated verbal labels. The play activities were of the toddler sort (e.g., fetching objects and putting them into, and taking them out of, containers and wagons). These activities offered many opportunities for naming and for discovering that the lexicalized categories were based on object shape. The experimenter would focus on one category at a time, each for five minutes. Two novel objects that differed in color and substance but were of the same shape, would be brought into the play activities and repeatedly given the same novel label (e.g., "We need a dax. Ah, here's a dax. Where's the other one?"). Also, an object that was not a category member would be introduced and identified as such, "*That's* not a _____." This basic format would then be repeated, with five minutes of play devoted in turn to each of the four types of objects.

Following the seven weeks of training, further probe testing indicated that the children would now extend the experiment nouns to new objects that were similar in shape, and more importantly, would use the same-shape strategy when responding to a brand new label. A group of age-matched controls showed neither of these abilities. Interestingly, the children who had received the language intervention still only knew about 26 count nouns. Apparently, their experiences in the focused training sessions had accelerated their learning of the shape bias, in effect substituting for the more haphazard experiences of everyday talk. If, as theorists believe, the same-shape strategy improves children's ability to determine the meaning of early nouns, these children should have been equipped to learn more words at an earlier age.

These studies by Linda Smith and her colleagues have two direct applications to clinical practice, one for children at the early stages of language learning and one for clients of all ages.

Learning to Learn

For as long as I can remember, the literature on language intervention has admonished us to teach children *how* to learn language rather than to merely teach them particular forms. Although this sounds like an excellent goal, no one, to my knowledge, has told us what the relevant learning processes are, nor how to foster them.

Thinking About Child Language

The Smith (2001) studies begin to fill in this gap, by implying that we can help children acquire the same-shape strategy. Armed with this strategy, children should be able to learn early nouns more easily.

The key elements in the Smith (2001) intervention program would seem to be (1) its focus and (2) its careful manipulation of context, both verbal and nonverbal. First, let's think about focus. Instead of the traditional approach of teaching the labels for several new words at the same time, each new object class and its label was introduced in a separate five-minute module. This made it possible for the therapist to use the new word at a very high proportional frequency, while the child was attending to members of the reference class of objects.

Even more than focus, however, I think it was the manipulation of the context which made this intervention successful. Object labels are not names. They apply to large, even infinitely large, sets of objects. In these training sessions, instead of playing with one instance of an object class, children played with two instances of the same shape but differing in size and color. They also saw the interventionist reject a third object that was not the same shape although it shared a property with the other two. Thus the *nonverbal* context provided powerful cues to the fact that the new word was the label for a class of objects rather than a proper noun, and further that members of the class could be identified by shape. If we were to do the same thing with real world objects, we might play with a large red rubber ball, a small blue sponge ball, and reject a small red metal car.

The *verbal* context was likewise manipulated. Children repeatedly heard phrases such as "I need the _____" or "Look, here's the _____." This, of course, provided children with repeated examples of the new noun. It also provided repeated examples of the carrier phrase that Smith believes to be the eventual key to the learning of the same-shape strategy.

Finally, note that the session included four identical modules, each with its own word and each crafted with the same attention to focus, object sets, and language framework. Any one of the modules could give the child knowledge of its particular word, but more than one module was needed if the child was to make the higher-level, learning-to-learn deduction that shape is the critical feature of lexicalized object classes. It is exactly because the child was drawn to the shape feature in a *succession* of modules, that the naming phrases could become associated with the notion of shape—a notion that was constant across the set. Once this has occurred, whenever a child hears "Look, here is a _____," he or she can immediately attend to the shape of the object and see it as a member of a lexicalized class.

The Developmental Model

Another intervention issue on which there has been much written is the relevance of "the normal model." Again we find two prevailing opinions. Many of the theorists working within the framework of behaviorism argue that the developmental patterns seen in normal children cannot provide relevant guidelines for intervention because children with language impairments are *not* normal learners. Other theorists, including myself, are more impressed by the essential normalcy of the language learning process, even for children for whom language is difficult. Their learning may be slow and effortful, but the fundamental relationships governing the emergence of language still seem to hold true. This is seen most clearly in the fact that patterns of language growth within the various linguistic domains (i.e., morphology, syntax, semantics) follow the same course of development for impaired learners as for children who are normal learners. But these fundamental relationships are also seen in the predictable language patterns that result from dysfunctions in cognition, perception, or emotional health. Slow conceptual development is reflected in late learning of relational terms; deficits in attention are reflected in late learning of grammatical morphology; inadequate theory of mind is reflected in inappropriate patterns of language use, and so forth.

At first read, the Smith (2001) studies seem to say that the facts of normal development can be easily altered. It is true that the same-shape strategy is usually learned at about 20 months and only after children know 50 count nouns. It is also true that the children in the training study were only 17 months of age and knew only 25 count nouns, and nevertheless acquired the same-shape learning strategy after only 2 hours and 20 minutes of teaching. I think, though, that in this case and many others, the deviation from the normal model lies only in the surface facts, not the underlying dependencies.

Think for a moment about the prerequisite knowledge, processes, and experience that might be needed in order to discover that shape is the key to learning count nouns. The cognitive requirements for the shape bias would be that children be capable of associative learning and able to perceive shape similarity. The first of these is present at birth and the second is acquired during the first year of life. What children need in addition is enough of the right kind of experience to discover that shape is important when trying to figure out what a new word means. Everyday conversations provide this experience only sporadically, and over great time intervals. Carefully crafted lessons compress this experience, highlighting the key variable. Basically, the training study accelerated acquisition of the shape strategy by improving the quality of experience, and this was possible exactly because the required cognitive abilities were available.

Whenever prerequisite knowledge and process is available, we can accelerate learning by changing the quality of the child's experience. This is what we do every day in language therapy. The result may change the superficial facts of language development, but not the underlying dependencies among schemes and processes.

Older Children

It is unlikely that we would be teaching the shape strategy to anyone over the mental age of 3. However, the general character of Smith's intervention program can guide us in developing programs for older children as well. While talking with a student about memory strategies this week I remembered (!) a study done 25 years ago by Ross and Ross (1978) that looked at 9-year-old children with global delays. At that time many researchers in the field of special education were investigating the role of memory deficits in mental retardation and there had been several unsuccessful attempts to teach the use of memory strategies. The training program developed by Ross and Ross was the first to succeed. What distinguished their program from the others was its *repeated* use of the same memory strategy in *a series* of *different games*. As was true for Smith, this program feature made it possible for children to distinguish the higher-level cognitive strategy from its use in a particular activity.

Caveat

We don't know whether the toddlers in the third Smith (2001) study did in fact learn words faster and earlier because they had acquired the same-shape strategy at a younger than normal age. We do know that strategies of this sort are reliably used by young children when learning new words in a laboratory setting, and it is easy to imagine that they would be useful as everyday tools as well. This is a good enough bet that if I were working with children at the early one-word stage, I would try Linda's training program. I will also be looking for further longitudinal studies of learning to learn. Clinical research on this topic would be particularly useful since looking at the acquisition of the same-shape strategy in older preschoolers with language impairment could help us understand the ways in which this strategy is tied to prior language knowledge and experience.❖

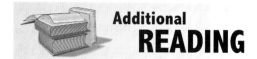

Additional
READING

Ross, D., & Ross, S. (1978). Facilitative effect of mnemonic strategies on multiple-associate learning in EMR children. *American Journal of Mental Deficiency, 82,* 460–466.

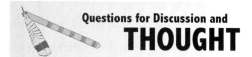

Questions for Discussion and
THOUGHT

1. Smith and her colleagues taught 17-month-old toddlers who knew only 26 words a strategy that normally is not acquired until children have learned 50 words. This suggests that "50 words" is not really a prerequisite for the same-shape strategy. Does this mean there is no prerequisite? Or is there a hidden variable here?

2. How would you adapt the same-shape strategy intervention for a child who is learning language with an AAC system?

3. Why do children stop using the same-shape strategy in the later preschool years?

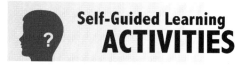

Self-Guided Learning
ACTIVITIES

1. **Try with toddlers.** Prepare materials so that you can test a child's knowledge of the same-shape strategy. You will need three sets of three unfamiliar objects. In each set two objects are the same shape, but different in size or color; the third object shares size or color but is a different shape. Play with each set for three minutes. Remember to use a repetitive phrase such as, "Look, here's a____" and "I need a _____," and also to reject the third object at some point. Once the materials are ready and you've practiced a bit, add

this test to your assessment battery. For any child whose language and/or communication skills resemble those of a two-year-old, present three trials of Smith's task to see if the child uses a shape strategy for choosing the new referent. What pattern emerges from children with language delays? Does the strategy seem to be linked to vocabulary size as expected?

2. **Try with school-age children.** Select a child whose learning targets include either (1) metacommunication strategies (e.g., requesting that instructions be repeated), or (2) memory strategies (e.g., rehearsal). Review your intervention activities. Do you use a wide enough range of examples to allow for generalization? Add more if needed.

Exploring the Scope of Language Intervention

I n my personal version of speech-language pathology, the focus of intervention is not just on the language system itself, as marvelous as that may be, but on language as the product and the servant of the mind. For me, language connects to everything—reason, social relationship, culture, learning, and reflection. The world of the clinician is not the world of linguists, or of psychologists, but the world of people—in our case, young people. Scientists have the luxury of studying narrow topics in great depth, but they sometimes miss the connections. The world of the child is all about connections. Not words for words' sake, but words in order to think, make friends, and learn about the world.

When you view language intervention this way, you worry less about your job description and professional territoriality, and more about acquiring and maintaining the breadth of knowledge needed for effective practice. The essays in this section represent just a few of the places I have discovered on my path of learning. They give some idea of the variety and challenge inherent in our profession—a wide range of problems and procedures, and an even wider scope of inquiry.

25 Grammar Books

We are used to the idea that research *results* can help us design therapy programs. I suspect, however, that we don't pay enough attention to research *tasks and materials*. Some of them make excellent tools for teaching and learning language. Before I tell you about one such tool, I need to set the stage by talking a bit about parent education programs.

Can Parents Help?

There are surprisingly few studies of the effects of parent education programs on children's language development, and those that have been done have produced mixed findings. Given the widespread use of this approach and its potential economies, we need to have a better understanding of the factors that determine its efficacy. There are some indications that the outcomes may depend on the child's language level and the parents' language capabilities.

The study by Girolametto et al. (1996) is one of the few to show that a parent education program can improve the language of children with atypical development. This Toronto team taught parents to interact with young children in ways that could facilitate language learning (e.g., maintaining the child's topic or expanding the child's utterances). Since group meetings alone had failed to produce changes in an earlier study (Tannock & Girolametto, 1992), the researchers in this study also met individually with each parent to help select suitable vocabulary goals for each child. Parents and researchers then worked together to identify the everyday activities that would provide natural teaching and learning opportunities for the chosen words. By the end of the 10 weeks, children whose parents had participated in the educational program had learned twice as many targeted words as children in a control group. These results certainly support the use of parent-centered intervention programs. However, Girolametto and his colleagues caution readers that their study only included children at the one-word stage and only targeted vocabulary goals. Two other studies suggest that these facts are important.

In her University of British Colombia masters thesis research, Carmen Parsons (1991) measured the relative effects of two parent education programs— one with, and one without, an individualized component. Like the Toronto researchers, she found better outcomes when individualized goals and training sessions were included. Unlike the Toronto parents, however, parents in the UBC study selected syntactic and pragmatic goals as well as vocabulary goals, and this fact led Parsons to a second important finding. The greatest gains were made by children who were at lower language levels and whose learning goals were confined to vocabulary growth and increased verbal communication. Children at more advanced language levels whose goals included new syntactic and morphological forms showed less progress. Parents of these children indicated frustration with the program and felt they were unable to provide facilitative contexts for the selected grammatical forms. As Parsons notes, "The communication targets for the less advanced children were somehow inherently 'easier' for parents than many of the more advanced targets" (p. 139).

This possibility is echoed in the results from Fey et al. (1993). These researchers compared the effects of an individualized parent program to the effects of therapy provided by an SLP. All of the children were speaking in short phrases and sentences at the outset, and most of the goals were in the area of syntax. Children in both treatment programs made better progress than children in a no-treatment control group. And, you'll be relieved to know that, although group means did not differ a great deal, children directly taught by the SLP did make greater gains than the children who received only indirect service. More interesting for our purposes here is the fact that there was much wider variability among the children who had been taught by a parent. Some parents were apparently very effective language teachers and others were very ineffective. The researchers note further that, "parents learned and applied recasts early on but found them less appropriate to use as their children's language became increasingly complex" (p. 154). Both of these studies, then, suggest that higher-level and/or syntactic learning goals are difficult for some parents to address.

I think that the researchers got this one right. In every class I teach, there are some students who analyze language with insight and creativity and other students who are mystified. There may be even greater diversity in the language abilities of parents of children with language impairments. When Tallal et al. (2001) gave standardized language tests to family members who were the close relatives of children with SLI, some 31 percent of them showed language deficits. And Dale et al. (1998) report that genetic factors were responsible for 73 percent of the variance among two-year-olds with language delay. It seems that there are real differences in language ability among competent adult speakers, and that parents of children with language impairments may have their own language difficulties. This clearly creates a problem for parent-centered intervention. The metalinguistic processing required for syntactic and morphological targets may just be too much for some parents to handle.

A Study of Speech Acoustics

I have never before done research in the area of acoustics and probably never will again, but one of my projects is taking me down this path. The project explores the reasons that some children have difficulty learning English grammatical morphemes, asking in particular whether there are factors other than perceptual salience at work. One possibility is that children with low language proficiencies don't attend to English grammatical morphemes because these forms are not needed to convey basic propositional meanings. In a language such as German where these forms play a more important semantic role, children might have different priorities. If so, children with language impairments who are learning German should have less difficulty with grammatical morphemes, other things being equal. That last phrase is the sticker. Are grammatical morphemes in the two languages equally easy for children to notice and analyze?

With this question in mind, I am planning to tape-record mothers who are native speakers of either English or German as they read a story to their preschool-age child. Morphological segments will be isolated and properties such as amplitude and duration will be measured. This will help us decide whether grammatical morphemes in the two languages indeed have equivalent perceptual salience. If so, any differences in learning patterns would stem from other factors such as utility.

Now comes the fun part—and the point of this essay. I decided to focus our first analyses on past-tense forms. In order to elicit a large number of these forms in a short time, we took a children's book and rewrote the text so as to include the largest possible number of regular past-tense verb endings. Here's a sample of the text:

> Tommy grabb<u>ed</u> a big piece of red Playdoh.
>
> He push<u>ed</u> and push<u>ed</u> and pull<u>ed</u> and pull<u>ed</u>
>
> and toss<u>ed</u> it into the air.
>
> He made it nice and round.

Then he sprink<u>led</u> it with sugar,

cover<u>ed</u> it with yellow frosting,

and plopp<u>ed</u> some raisins on top.

Then Tommy went upstairs and said,

"Mommy, look! Daddy bak<u>ed</u> this cookie just for you."

You may recognize this as an adaptation of Robert Munsch's book *Mmm, Cookies!* (2000). As the story unfolds, Tommy fools different people with his Playdoh cookies, allowing the above excerpt to be repeated three times. The pictures are grand, and the topic is one that is sure to please preschool-age children.

As I was talking with my students about intervention this week, it struck me that this research tool would also be an excellent intervention tool. All in all, there are 66 past-tense endings in this story. Since the book takes about 4.5 minutes to read, the child is hearing 15 past-tense endings per minute. With the aid of this book, even parents who blanch at morphology would be able to provide focused stimulation for this grammatical goal. Moreover, repetitions within the text, combined with repetitive readings, should create good opportunities for parental scaffolding, where children could fill in the blanks with newly learned verb forms. And why stop with the past tense? I can easily envision a series of books, each highlighting a specific grammatical form or pattern. These texts would be easy to prepare, and once prepared could be sent home with family after family.

Will It Work?

The language used while reading books can be quite different than language used for other purposes. Highly familiar texts eventually become routinized and lose much of their communicative force. Also, forms learned in only one context may not be fully understood. In the case of the past tense, for example, it is unlikely that a child could learn either its perfective or its past-time meanings from hearing it used only in narratives. However, once a child has acquired a word or morpheme in a routine context, it can become an old form ready to acquire new functions as it is heard in everyday conversation.

A study by Yoder et al. (1995) lends some credibility to this line of thinking. Children with global developmental delays were enrolled in a book reading program. Each child participated in daily book reading sessions with an adult who asked questions about the story and then expanded the child's response utterances. Since the same book was used from day to day, sessions were highly repetitive and soon led to routinized exchanges. In comparison to a baseline, many of the children showed convincing gains in MLU during the two-month program. Interestingly, it was again children at lower language levels who showed the most gain. The researchers note that while they did not match their language models to the child's level, the session protocols in fact featured patterns that are typically learned by younger children. If they had used focused expansion of forms that were matched to the child's level, they might have seen gains in more advanced children as well.

The Yoder et al. (1995) study demonstrates that child-directed talk while book reading can be an effective source of information about language form, even for children who are slow learners. Many of my colleagues in British Columbia already use children's books as a general forum for parent-child interaction, and also recommend books that have repetitive language. I am intrigued by the idea that we could extend this practice to include focused models of particular grammatical forms. This could assist parents who find it difficult to facilitate the use of these forms in everyday conversation, and it also will be a welcome suggestion to busy parents who already read to their children regularly.❖

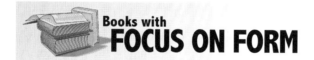

Books with FOCUS ON FORM

The Story Box. (Originally published by Ginn, now published by the Wright Group, www.wrightgroup.com.) See especially the books at the Emergent Reader level, which use predictable language. They are intended for early literacy, but may be easily used as suggested in this essay. The books contain colorful pictures and interesting content. Over 100 titles use repetitive language forms in specific books including question forms, pronouns, prepositions, and plurals. Higher-level books have simple play scripts which can be used with groups.

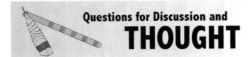

Questions for Discussion and
THOUGHT

1. The text of the story *Mmm, Cookies!* (Munsch, 2000) was changed to focus on regular past tense forms. Could you imagine changing other storybooks to focus on your current learning targets, or are there just certain forms that would be appropriate for this approach to intervention?

2. What are the qualities to look for in a children's storybook that you intend to alter in the fashion described in this essay?

3. What would you listen for as you talked to a child's parent in order to decide whether or not the parent had strong language skills? Are there questions you could ask that would help you with this decision?

4. While consulting with a parent, you notice that he or she doesn't speak very often and uses only simple sentences. This might indicate limitations in the parent's language skills, but there could be other reasons for this reticence. What other explanations should you consider?

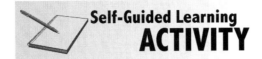

Self-Guided Learning
ACTIVITY

If you haven't already done so, answer questions 1 and 2 above. Then go to a children's bookstore and look for a storybook that you could alter for a particular client. Purchase the book. (If you get hooked on this idea, maybe the local Rotary Club would help you buy lots of books.) Then get creative and rewrite the text. Think about the mechanics a bit. I typed the new text on my computer, spacing it so I could tape the sheets right over the existing text. That way I can remove them and use the story again in a different fashion. Perhaps you can think of a better system.

26 One, Two, Buckle My Shoe

Tell me, Billy, how many pigs are there?

One, two, three, four, five, six, seven [pointing to each].

Right, so how many pigs are there?

One, two, three, four, five, six, seven [pointing to each].

OK, so how many pigs are there?

One, two, three, four, five, six, seven [pointing to each].

My conversation with this bright four-year-old really happened. As is very clear, Billy had not yet learned to use the last number word spoken to represent the number of objects in the set. Over the past two and a half decades, researchers have shown us that this is just one aspect of counting that children must learn. Before it can become a verbal yardstick for measuring quantities, children must (1) memorize the counting routine itself, (2) segment this rote material into separate quantity terms, and (3) learn how to place each term into one-to-one correspondence with the objects in a set. Only after these things are in place can children discover the principle of *cardinality,* that the furthest point in the counting routine can be used to ascertain and represent quantities.

An important feature of this developmental story is that different aspects of counting seem to draw on different strands of prior learning, and to involve somewhat different mental mechanisms. Initial learning of the sequence of number words requires good auditory memory for phonological strings and efficient, reliable access to those representations. The counting routine when first learned, however, has little or no linkage to quantification concepts. It takes on these meanings later as the child constructs higher-level quantification schemes out of his or her experiences with object sets.

In data from the Ottawa longitudinal study (Young et al., 2002), young adults who had been diagnosed with language impairments at age 5 are still having difficulties with mathematics at age 19. About 55 percent show significant delays in this area—more even than are having trouble with reading. We are used to thinking about the relationships between early language delays and later reading problems, but there has been little attention to the relationships between early language impairment and later problems with mathematics. However, a five-year longitudinal project designed and implemented by Barbara Fazio provides some important initial data.

When the Sound Stick Falters

Fazio conducted a series of studies that looked at the mathematical abilities of children with SLI. Fazio's first study (1994) looked at counting abilities in a group of 20 children with specific language impairments. These children were matched by mental age to a group of normally developing peers and to a group of children with mild retardation from the same schools. A third control group of younger, normally developing children were matched to the SLI children by language level, using scores derived from spontaneous language samples. All of the children performed the same set of experimental tasks: reciting number words, counting object sets, and learning and using a gestural counting scheme.

On the rote counting tasks, the children with SLI did much less well than the children in the two control groups. They recited fewer counting words, found them difficult to say backwards, and were less accurate when they were asked to count sets of objects. Interestingly, their errors tended to be errors in the order of the words rather than in one-to-one correspondences. The final two tasks involved cardinality judgments. Here the picture was somewhat different. Children in the SLI group could not answer quickly when asked how many, but when they did answer, they gave the last counting word spoken as their answer, thereby demonstrating their understanding of cardinality.

So far, these findings point to auditory memory rather than conceptualization as the source of the SLI children's mathematical difficulties. These children seem not to have been able to acquire the rote string of number words that serves as a fundamental measuring stick—or in this case a *sound stick*—for young children. To follow up on this possibility, Fazio collected data from another series of counting tasks, this time using a novel gestural counting routine. Children were taught to point to a sequence of body parts as an alternative to oral counting. Although the SLI children performed less well than their age peers when counting with the gesture system, they were nevertheless better at gesture counting than at oral counting. This finding is what would be expected from learners with deficits in the auditory processing of phonological representations. The group with mild mental retardation showed just the opposite profile, in accord with their slower rate of learning.

Two Years Later

Fazio (1996) was able to reassess most of the children in her SLI, language control, and MA control groups two years later, after they had completed two years of schooling. In addition to the counting tasks used earlier, Fazio asked the children to match sets by size, calculate the total number of objects across two sets, identify the larger of two sets, read and write numerals, and do simple addition problems (timed and untimed, written and oral).

Children in the SLI group now performed as well as their MA peers on the counting tasks, as long as the quantities did not exceed 10. They could likewise add object sets, and read and write numerals, as long as the quantities were small. However, in all of the addition calculations with number symbols rather than objects, the SLI group was less successful than the peer group and used less sophisticated strategies. For example, when adding 3 + 2, the MA controls would start with the larger quantity, 3, and just add 2 more, while the SLI children would start with 1.

Fazio notes that the children in the SLI group, given time, and quantities small enough to allow use of their fingers, were quite good at solving the addition problems with objects. In this regard, they outperformed younger children at the same language levels, and showed knowledge of basic mathematical concepts and procedures. However, counting larger quantities was still a challenge for the SLI children and they were not memorizing the math facts that make rapid calculations possible (e.g., that 6 + 3 = 9 or 7 + 4 = 11). This failure again seems to implicate auditory memory processes. As mathematical calculations become more complex, lack of access to memorized material could impede higher-level conceptual learning.

Five Years Later

In the latest installment to this series, Fazio (1999) reports on the progress of this group of SLI children when they reach grades 4 and 5. The demands of the mathematics curriculum at this level are considerable: multidigit addition, subtraction, and multiplication; math fact retrieval; long division; the use of fractions; and concepts related to money. The language needed for discussing these concepts and procedures is complex, including terms such as *divisor* or *denominator,* and children increasingly meet the dreaded word problem. There would seem to be plenty of challenge for children who have difficulty processing language and accessing memorized material.

This time Fazio gave the children a series of written arithmetic problems, ingeniously disguised as an adventure comic book, as well as a standardized math test. The arithmetic problems were given both timed and untimed. Children with SLI did less well than their normally developing age peers in all tasks, but three findings stand out as particularly interesting. First, the children with SLI did significantly better on the arithmetic problems in the untimed condition, while the normally developing children showed no difference between timed and untimed performance. Second, scores on a test of language comprehension and on a digit recall task were strongly correlated with math fact knowledge, and with speed and accuracy of written calculation in the timed condition. Finally, scores on the math facts task correlated strongly, but negatively, with speed of written calculation (i.e., children who had trouble retrieving math fact knowledge took more time to calculate).

Language and Math

Fazio's findings shed much light on the Ottawa longitudinal data (Young et al; 2002). The auditory rote memory difficulties that were first seen in preschoolers who couldn't count are seen later in older school-age children who can't remember their math facts. If the mind were not a limited capacity system, this memory problem wouldn't matter. The child or adult could merely figure out the components of the problem one more time, from scratch. In a limited capacity system, however, speed does make a difference and mental energy spent in redoing basic calculations is energy that is not available for more complex mathematical reasoning. The point of Fazio's work is not that SLI children need more time to complete their math problems, but that poor access to stored mathematical information impedes arithmetic calculation, and ultimately affects learning. The SLI children in Fazio's study are already a year behind their peers in mathematics by grades 4 to 5, and the Ottawa data suggest that this gap will increase with age.

This is a different view of the relationship between language impairment and difficulty with mathematics. We are used to thinking about the demands of word problems or the meanings of mathematical terms. We've read articles about "Language and the Curriculum" and understand the need to prepare language-impaired children with the vocabulary they will need to follow instructional discourse. We may even be counseling teachers to provide visual cues to word problems for children who are poor language processors. Fazio's data point in an additional direction. For her, the link between language and mathematics resides in the cognitive mechanisms that underlie activities in both of these domains. Many children with specific language impairments have been shown to have limitations in auditory memory. These limitations most probably affect language learning and use; Fazio's work now indicates that they also affect progress in mathematical reasoning.

Memory Lessons or Keypads?

As those of us who have reached middle age know all too well, memory problems are not easy to ameliorate. Fazio suggests a number of intervention strategies and notes that we may need to implement all of them at once. First, drill and practice on counting routines and math facts will definitely improve memory access. The challenge here is to make the exercises entertaining enough that children will not abandon mathematics all together. Computer games would seem to be the best bet for such practice. Second, extra time spent reviewing math concepts, terms, and procedures will leave children less vulnerable to error when a math fact needs to be recovered. We can incorporate such review into our sessions, or check to ensure that some other member of the educational team is doing so. Finally, some experts in mathematics instruction have offered the heretical idea that the use of calculators is not all bad. As Fazio concludes, once a child demonstrates fundamental understanding of a given concept or operation, use of a calculator may be an entirely appropriate accommodation for slow computation. It may take some time, however, to demonstrate to teachers that a child's mathematical errors are due to slow or faulty retrieval of counting routines and math facts, rather than poor conceptualization. Some of us may even need to brush up on our own mathematical understandings before we can do so.❖

Thinking About Child Language

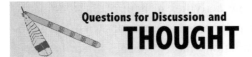

Questions for Discussion and
THOUGHT

1. Fazio argues that language and mathematics are related because both rely on auditory working memory, especially in the early stages of learning. From other sources, we know that these two areas are also related because mathematics has a unique vocabulary which requires some degree of prior knowledge before the words can be learned. And finally, the two areas are clearly related because counting words are the first tool for unitized quantification. If we take this domain as a mental microcosm, we could conclude that language depends on thought, that thought depends on language, and that both depend on a third factor. How do we make sense of this? Do all domains show this same set of diverse influences? Is there any point in talking about what comes first?

2. Where are the best points for SLP intervention in arithmetic learning, if any?

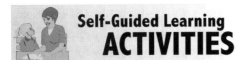

Self-Guided Learning
ACTIVITIES

1. **Try with preschool children.** Fazio mentions three behavioral tests of early quantification: rote recitation of number words; pointing to each object in a set and saying one of the number words individually and in order; and answering the cardinality question by repeating the last number reached in the counting. Predict how each four-year-old on your caseload will handle each of these tasks, then confirm your predictions with some data! Be sure to notice what sorts of errors are made. Do the results indicate differences among the children? Do some children count accurately, but don't seem to know how to *use* the sound stick? Do other children make counting errors and fail to come up with the right answer, but nevertheless convince you that they understand set quantification? What is the key evidence of advanced conceptualization?

2. **Try with school-age children.** Check on the math achievement levels of the children on your caseload who are in grades 3 or 4. If they are having difficulty, ask their teachers about the possibility of access to computerized practice on math facts. If the school doesn't have software of this sort, investigate and recommend. Try www.superkids.com for educational software reviews.

27 The Best Route to Reading

The Reading Debate

No educational debate is longer, more fractious, or less resolved than the debate over reading instruction. For decades, Phonics and Basic Skills approaches of one sort or another have been pitted against Language Experience and Whole Language approaches, in recurrent cycles that have more to do with politics, economics, and belief than with learning theory. SLPs have an increasing stake in these debates. We now know that most four-year-olds with specific language impairments will have difficulties learning to read. Families and schools want our advice about how to assist these children. Moreover, SLPs who work in schools are themselves likely to be involved in reading instruction as tutors or consultants, especially given the current enthusiasm for phonological awareness training. What is most wrong-headed about the ongoing debate is the tendency to treat literacy learning and reading instruction in either-or terms. A study by Catts et al. (1999) provides compelling evidence that educators have been fighting a false battle.

A Longitudinal, Large-Sample Study of Reading and Reading Disabilities

Catts et al. (1999) was designed to evaluate the relative importance of phonological processing and oral language abilities in literacy learning. The evaluation was done in two ways: by comparing the kindergarten test profiles of good and poor readers in grade 2, and by looking to see whether kindergarten phonological and oral language scores would predict grade 2 reading achievement.

Certain features of the Catts et al. (1999) project make their findings particularly believable. First, the data are longitudinal, with a large battery of test scores for each child at both kindergarten and grade 2. Second, the sample includes children with a wide range of cognitive abilities. Many prior studies have excluded children with below-average IQ. Since most IQ tests are heavily dependent on verbal abilities, this has, in effect, excluded children with language disorders and biased the results. Third, the study was designed such that the results are representative of children from varied economic, cultural, and educational backgrounds. Finally, the study measures the relationships between reading achievement and *both* phonological abilities and oral language abilities. It thus can weigh the relative importance of prior learning in these two areas. Now let's look at the study outcomes.

The first analysis compared the kindergarten test profiles of children who were good and poor readers in grade 2. Out of the 604 children who participated, there were 183 children who were identified as poor readers, with scores on a grade 2 reading comprehension battery at least 1 *SD* below the mean. The remaining children were considered good readers. The researchers compared the test scores of these two groups of children when they were in kindergarten, looking at phonological awareness, rapid naming, picture vocabulary, oral vocabulary, sentence comprehension, sentence imitation, morphosyntax, and narrative. These basic test scores were combined in various ways to yield scores for vocabulary, grammar, narrative, receptive language, and expressive language. Additionally, at grade 2 there were tests of word recognition and verbal/nonverbal intelligence. Some of the major findings are shown in the chart below:

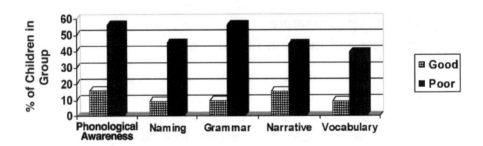

Kindergarten Scores of Grade 2 Good and Poor Readers: % Children below -1 *SD*

Children who were poor readers in grade 2 were much more likely to have had deficits (more than 1 *SD* below the mean) in phonological processing and/or oral language abilities in kindergarten than children who were good readers. Deficits in oral language were as common as deficits in phonological processing, and while the two sorts of deficit often occurred in combination, they also occurred alone at equivalent rates. Interestingly, the overall pattern of results was not much different when the poor readers were defined by word recognition rather than comprehension tests.

The second analysis looked to see whether phonological processing and oral language scores would predict grade 2 reading achievement. Multiple regression is a statistical procedure that looks simultaneously at the correlations among a set of variables and compares their relative predictive strength. When Catts and his colleagues analyzed their data in this fashion, they found that oral language skills in kindergarten were a better predictor of grade 2 *reading comprehension* than were phonological processing skills, although each of these two areas of ability had reliable value as a predictor. When they analyzed the data again to see which variables would predict grade 2 *word recognition,* oral language and phonological processing abilities were equally good predictors, and again each of the two areas were shown to have independent and reliable predictive value.

Oral Language and Literacy

As researchers always say, these are only correlational data and cannot prove causal connections. However, keeping in mind that these correlations come from longitudinal data and can be readily interpreted within theories of literacy, I believe they do point to factors that fundamentally influence reading success. SLPs should especially note the clear connection between oral language ability and later reading achievement. There are two ways to look at this correlation. It could reflect common aspects of the two learning tasks. Whatever cognitive processes are involved in learning to speak could also be involved in learning to read. If so, children with processing limitations that hindered their oral language learning would also be hindered in literacy learning. Alternatively, the correlation could reflect the fact that reading is not merely a decoding skill, but is a mode of meaningful verbal communication. Reading processes thus utilize the same stored language knowledge that is used in oral language, and children who arrive with delays in oral language development will be impoverished readers, lacking the grammatical knowledge and vocabulary knowledge needed to interpret the printed text.

It seems likely to me that both of these interpretations are true. As SLPs, we can help children learn more about language before they enter school, and thus ensure that they will have more resource knowledge to use in learning to read. However, whatever basic processing deficits exist may be less amenable to therapy.

Assessing Reading Success

The second thing to notice about these findings is that the nature of the best predictor depended on how reading was defined. If word recognition (e.g., word calling, reading single words aloud) is taken as the index of literacy, then phonological processing is a good predictor of success. But if, instead, we look at reading comprehension as the index of literacy, then oral language abilities are a better predictor of success. It is important to keep this in mind as we evaluate the claims of the many remedial reading programs now on the market. Although phonological processing skills are useful tools in cracking the written code, they are just a small part of the language knowledge that most children bring to literacy learning. Improvement in phonological awareness may lead to better word recognition, but it may not be sufficient to guarantee improvement in reading comprehension.

Back to the Debate

Armed with knowledge of the Catts et al. (1999) study, we may be able to influence the ongoing debate about reading instruction as it plays out in our home communities. As I suggested in the opening paragraph, this debate has been too simple for too long. The Catts data indicate clearly that reading success has at least two independent roots—phonological processing *and* oral language abilities. Our colleagues on school boards and curriculum committees don't need to choose between phonics and language experience approaches to reading instruction. They need rather to create opportunities for both sorts of literacy learning. As acknowledged experts in language development, we may be able to help public educators reframe the issues.❖

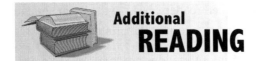 **Additional READING**

Catts, H., Fey, M., & Zhang, X. (2001). Estimating the risk of future reading difficulties in kindergarten children: A research-based model and its clinical implementation. *Language, Speech, and Hearing Services in Schools 32*, 38–50.

Swanson, L., Trainin, F., & Necoechea, D. (2003). Rapid naming, phonological awareness, and reading: A meta-analysis of the correlation evidence. *Review of Educational Research, 73*, 407–440.

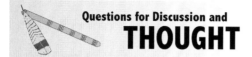

1. How does oral language knowledge influence the reading process for beginning readers?

2. Some children with severe language learning impairments seem to gain their initial language knowledge by reading, instead of by speaking. Do these children contradict the Catts et al. (1999) findings?

3. Why does the primary school curriculum place such emphasis on reading aloud?

4. Imagine a child in grade 1 who has a history of language delay, but has had SLP services as a preschooler and now speaks quite well, albeit more simply than his or her age peers. This child's parents are now concerned about the fact that he or she is having trouble with reading. Is there any value in talking with them about the connections between oral language delays and reading problems? If so, what would be your main points?

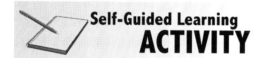

Self-Guided Learning
ACTIVITY

Find out which tests are being used in your school district to evaluate reading success in grades 1 and 2. Look at the items on these tests and determine how many require only word recognition skills and how many require comprehension skills. Do the proportions change with grade level? Now pay attention to the nature of the task that is used to determine either word recognition or comprehension. Could children have some knowledge of the word and still fail the task? How could you find out?

28 Sharing Our Knowledge

Early in my clinical career, I attended a conference for preschool interventionists that was sponsored by parents. There were the usual presentations by experts, but the session that really caught my attention was one featuring a panel of parents whose children had been diagnosed with developmental disorders. I will never forget their two main messages to the professionals in the audience that day.

First, they wanted us to understand and remember that while each of us was completely centered on our particular area of treatment (e.g., speech and language or gross motor skills), they had a broader perspective. We might believe that the sign for *more* was the most important goal for the week, but they had jobs, cared for entire families, and could not possibly put top priority on the recommendations of each of the professionals they dealt with. They respected our in-depth expertise, but we in turn needed to respect the constant juggling of people and tasks that was their everyday challenge.

Second, these parents asked us to give them the same time to learn that we give their children. What a simple and profound request. We don't expect new words to be fully acquired after a single hearing, or the plural to be mastered after one practice session. We recognize that new language representations and new concepts take time to construct and even more time to integrate with prior knowledge. This is especially true when existing frameworks must change to accommodate the new learning. What we sometimes forget is that these expectations for therapy outcomes reflect general principles of learning that apply to adults as well as to children. Too often, we schedule a single conference, make our pronouncements, and expect parents to understand.

I was reminded of this conference when I read the report of a recent survey conducted by the Canadian organization Invest in Kids (Oldershaw, 2002). The project was designed to find out what parents knew about development and what they believed about parenting. The findings were sobering.

A National Survey of Parents of Young Children

Participating parents were selected on the basis of their child's date of birth. Only households with children under age 6 were selected. The survey questions were designed by child development experts, but the other aspects of the study were conducted by a commercial survey firm. The sampling was done in two stages to insure that it approximated the demographics of Canadian society in regard to parental age, sex, marital status, province, population density, language, and household income. Some 1,640 surveys were ultimately returned for analysis (a 38 percent return rate) and sampling error was estimated at 2.4 percent.

Views on the Importance of Parenting

Survey results indicated that 92 percent of Canadian parents think that parenting is the most important thing they can do, and 94 percent enjoy being a parent most of the time. Some 79 percent of parents agreed strongly that the years from ages 0 to 5 are critical to the way "a child turns out as an adult" and, moreover, 84 percent strongly agreed that parental influence during those years was a crucial determinant of developmental outcomes.

Self-Reports of Parenting Behaviors

A set of questions concerning parenting behaviors was used to statistically generate three parenting dimensions: positive/warm interactions, angry and punitive parenting, and ineffective child management. Although the majority of parents scored on the positive end of these dimensions, some did not. Thirty-four percent judged themselves to be ineffective in child management, and 36 percent reported that they did not have warm interactions with their children. Sixty-two percent said that they regularly use punitive/angry behaviors when their children misbehave, and half of the parents reported at least occasional physical punishment.

Knowledge about Child Development

The survey also included true/false questions about early developmental achievements and the role of the environment in supporting children's growth. I'll list them here without the answers so you can check your own knowledge. The figures in parentheses indicate the percentage of parents who answered correctly.

1. Babies are learning from the moment they are born. (94)

2. Parents' emotional closeness with their baby can strongly influence that child's intellectual development. (73)

3. The things a child experiences before the age of 3 will greatly influence his or her ability to do well in school. (52)

4. If a baby does not receive appropriate stimulations (e.g., being read to, played with, or touched and held) his or her brain will not develop as well as the brain of a baby who does receive these types of stimulation. (63)

5. Every baby is born with a certain level of intelligence which cannot be either increased or decreased by how parents interact with him or her. (44)

6. The more stimulation babies receive by holding and talking to them, the more you spoil them (60).

7. A baby can't communicate much until he or she is able to speak at least a few words. (59)

8. The average 1-year-old can say one or two words, but understands many more words and phrases. (54)

9. One-year-olds often cooperate and share when they play together. (26)

10. Intellectual development is the most important part of a child's being ready for school. (14)

11. By age 1, a baby's brain is fully developed. (38)

Some of these questions could have been worded more clearly, but even taking this into account it would seem that many Canadian parents are not well informed about aspects of early development that would affect everyday interactions with their children.

How well did you do? The answers are at the end of the essay. I should also explain that parents answered these questions on a scale from 0 (disagree completely) to 10 (agree completely). The authors counted only those answers at the extremes of the scale (i.e., 0 or 10) as being correct, but this seemed unreasonable to me given the complexity of the issues, so I counted 0–1 or 9–10 as being correct. The percentages listed above are thus somewhat larger than those given in the report.

Confidence in Parenting Skills

A further section of the survey asked parents to indicate how confident they were about their parenting skills and how their level of confidence might have changed over time. Prior to the birth of their first child, 44 percent of the respondents felt confident of their parenting skills. Not surprisingly, this level of confidence plummeted to 15 percent shortly after their first child was born. It eventually rises again, but no higher than 43 percent overall. Many parents remain unsure of how to handle difficult situations with their child, find it hard to understand their child's feelings and needs, or in general question their ability to parent.

Emotional Well-Being and Support

The final sections of the survey concerned the parents' own emotional health and their sources of support. Here the facts are disturbing. Forty-eight percent of single mothers, 28 percent of married mothers, and 19 percent of married fathers reported symptoms of depression on a standardized depression scale. About 40 percent of the parents reported disagreements with their spouse about child rearing practices, and 56 percent felt that their spouses should help more with parental responsibilities. Almost half of the parents agreed that they were "constantly under stress trying to accomplish more than I can handle," and 58 percent were spending less time with their children than they would like. To find help with these challenges, parents turned to pediatricians, spouses or partners, friends, their own mothers, and books/magazines (but only infrequently).

The overall picture that emerges from this survey is at one level familiar and predictable. Parents believe in the importance of their role, but feel uncertain of their abilities. They often lack the knowledge they need to make good parenting decisions, and experience considerable levels of stress stemming from busy lives and parental duties. At another level, however, what struck me in this report was the numbers. How could 74 percent of the parents expect one-year-olds to play cooperatively, or 36 percent experience no warm interaction with their children? What is the cost to society when 57 percent of parents feel incompetent for a life task they clearly value?

And What Does Any of This Have to Do with Speech-Language Pathology?

The answer to this question will, to some degree, depend upon our understanding of the nature of SLP services. For those of us who practice as professional experts, these findings invite restraint in judging parents as either supporting or hindering our treatment programs. Instead, we can respect their commitment to parenting and provide new information that will improve their confidence and decision-making abilities—always remembering the advice of the panel that has resonated in my mind for so many years: "Give us time."

For those of us who practice in a collaborative, family-centered fashion, this report may at first seem quite challenging since it reveals more needs than strengths. But, in the words of one advocate (Kwok, 2002), "Family-centered intervention firmly believes that all families have strengths and inherent abilities to develop competencies. Therefore, all professional interventions have to be tailored to ensure optimum opportunities for families to develop and strengthen their capabilities and competence in working with the child" (p. 7). What a greatly optimistic viewpoint! And one that the panel would have appreciated.

But all of this is just a fine tuning of business as usual. More importantly, these survey data invite us to Think Big. The fact is that most of us invest our energies in the service of a small number of children with developmental disabilities. Maybe the time has come to look beyond our caseloads to the community at large. As I read the report I couldn't help but realize that I knew the answers to virtually all of the questions about child development, and I suspect that most of you did as well. How can we share this knowledge with more families, even those whose children are developing normally? Perhaps we can join with early childhood educators and other professionals to offer community-based classes, newsletters, or websites that would be child development resources for all parents. The report suggests that this would be another, increasingly important, direction for SLP services to take. It may not be in your current job description, but it could be!❖

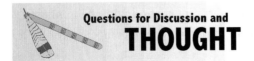

Questions for Discussion and
THOUGHT

1. What are the most important things about child development that parents need to understand in order to be effective partners in your intervention program? What do you do now, and what could you do, in order to help them learn these things?

2. There is little evidence that parents are causal factors in developmental language disorders, but there is evidence that they are key determinants of intervention outcomes—especially their attitudes towards their children. Are there ways we can help parents of children with communication disorders feel more positive about their children?

3. Does your job description allow you to spend time in preventative activities, such as speaking with parent groups or teacher groups about language development and disorders? What is your reaction to the proposal that SLPs should broadly share our knowledge rather than just treat individual children?

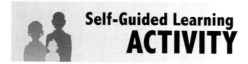

Self-Guided Learning
ACTIVITY

How and when do the young parents in your community learn about child development? Are courses on this topic required in the high school curriculum? Are there workshops offered in maternity hospitals? Prenatal classes in public health units? Make some phone calls and create a list of community resources for young parents. Think about how and what you could contribute to the programs that you discover.

Survey Answers: (1) T (2) T (3) T (4) T (5) F (6) F (7) F (8) T (9) F (10) F (11) F

29 Animal Charades

Language therapists started using sign language with children who could both speak and hear in the late 1960s. I remember thinking at the time that ASL would certainly be more convenient than the 3 × 5 cards and felt pens that I carried around with me so as to be able to create visual support for language learning. Events intervened, and I moved on to doctoral studies before I learned to sign. I remained curious, however, about the effects of this intervention strategy.

While working for a large California school district, I had the opportunity to visit a class of preschoolers with language impairments whose teacher (an SLP) had been using simultaneous sign and speech for six months. As we chatted about her experiences, I was interested to learn that she was going to abandon her use of sign in the classroom. She had kept no hard data, but her explanation made sense. Over the six months she had been using "total communication" (i.e., sign and speech), she had seen two types of changes in the children: their spoken language had greatly improved, and they no longer watched her sign. Initially the children had known very little oral language, and sign language had apparently provided important cues to both form and meaning. Although she never required it, the children had always stopped what they were doing and watched her when she spoke and signed. Now they didn't, and judging from their success in following directions, this was because they now could understand her speech. The teacher felt that the children themselves were telling her that sign language had been, but was no longer, necessary.

Using Signs for Speech

Until recently, my thinking on this topic had changed very little since visiting that classroom. My reading had led me to an initial understanding of two situations in which sign language could be used to good advantage with children who could speak and hear. First, for children with auditory perceptual problems, simultaneous sign and speech can provide better access to spoken language. Sign language presents a static, visual-spatial version of what is otherwise a rapidly changing, auditory-temporal event. For children with information processing difficulties, the stable nature of signs makes them easier to identify than spoken words. As instances of a given sign recur, children can recognize them as being the same. This allows them to identify analogous similarities in the accompanying spoken words despite having perceived them less accurately or fully.

Second, for some children with global developmental delays, signs seem easier to learn than spoken words. One explanation for this fact draws on the literature dealing with the development of imitative skills. Bates (1979) identifies imitation skills as one of three prerequisites to first words, and this is not hard to accept. Children clearly must be able to reproduce the sound strings they hear in order to speak. But what about gestures? Piaget (1962) argued that the first success in replicating novel actions occurs with hand and arm gestures because children can see these actions on their own bodies and can directly compare their own movement and configuration patterns to those of the model. There is no need for cross-modal transfer. Imitating novel sounds, in contrast, requires the infant to translate a visual-auditory event into a kinesthetic-auditory event. The fact that sign gestures can likewise be seen on one's own hands should make them easier to imitate than sound strings, and ultimately should make sign symbols easier to learn than vocal symbols.

This prediction has been confirmed by Goodwyn and Acredolo (1993), who demonstrated that gesture symbols are indeed learned at younger ages and more easily than their spoken counterparts. Together these lines of evidence suggest that children who are slow learners could develop a small repertory of signs to use while they are acquiring speech. At the very least, such interim use of sign could improve communication and reduce frustration for children and families. As we will see in a moment, this is just the beginning of the story.

More Gestures, More Talk

Despite these good arguments, many parents reject the use of ASL or gesture symbols because they fear that these systems will interfere with learning to speak. A recent report by Goodwyn et al. (2000) should help to allay these fears. These researchers involved 103 infants in a longitudinal study of the effects of gesture use. Participants were divided into three groups. In the Sign Training group (N = 32) parents were taught methods for promoting the use of symbolic gestures by their children. The key idea was to pair simple gestures with words (e.g., flapping their arms while saying "birdie" or sniffing while saying "flower." I was reminded here of my niece who absolutely adored animal charades.) In the Verbal Training group (N = 32) parents were encouraged to promote oral language development by labeling objects in context. To get things rolling for both intervention groups, five symbols were selected as initial intervention targets and parents were given books that contained many pictures of the referents for these words or gestures. In the Nonintervention Control group (N = 39) parents received no instruction at all and were not even told that the study focused on language development.

The children were 11 months old when the study began and all were developing normally. The groups were initially matched for income, parental education, birth order, gender, frequency of vocalization, and size of comprehension vocabulary. Children were retested at 15, 19, 24, 30, and 36 months of age. The assessment sessions included a video-taped play episode at 24 months (to determine frequency of vocalization, MLU, longest utterance), and a standardized-test battery at each data point (SICD, CDI, receptive and expressive single word vocabulary tests, and a test of phoneme discrimination). In addition, parents were interviewed every two weeks by telephone and reported the frequency with which the symbols had been modeled, and the frequency with which they had been used by the child. If a child was reported to be using a symbol, the nature of that use was explored in-depth to determine whether there was generalized use (multiple referents and a variety of communicative purposes) or context-bound use (a single referent and purpose). Only the former usage was considered to be truly symbolic.

Preliminary analyses indicated that the Sign Training had been effective. Children in that group acquired an average of 20 symbolic gestures while children in earlier studies without intervention had acquired on average only 5 symbolic gestures. The toddlers learned gesture symbols for such meanings as *drink, more, monkey, water, pig, giraffe, fish, smelly,* and *out.*

Preliminary analyses also indicated that children in the Verbal Training group did *not* have higher language scores at any point than did the children in the Control group, who were not receiving any intervention at all. Apparently, the testing sessions, phone calls, and parental focus on language development were by themselves not sufficient to accelerate language learning.

Results for the Sign Training group were dramatically different. At all testing points, language scores for children in the Sign Training group were higher than those for children in the Control group. Group differences during the second year (i.e., at 15, 19, and 24 months) were the largest, and many of them were statistically reliable. This was true for receptive and expressive vocabulary measures and for syntax measures drawn from the video-taped play session at 24 months. Instead of interfering, it seemed that early gesture symbols had actually led to an acceleration of spoken language development.

Rethinking Signs

As you can imagine, the Goodwyn et al. (2000) study generated considerable discussion among educators and theorists. As I sifted through the various arguments, I came to a better understanding of the ways that gesture symbols can facilitate language learning. The children in this study were neither perceptually impaired nor developmentally delayed. Yet, early training in the use of sign symbols led to early advances in language. Drawing on their interview data and findings from earlier studies, the researchers point to three sources for this effect. First, "the more things a child can and does talk about, the more vocal language the child will hear in return" (p. 99). Parents and other caregivers readily respond to toddlers' first efforts to communicate, and they most often respond with speech. "Doggie? Yes, that's a doggie. He's wagging his tail." Since gesture symbols tend to be learned earlier than vocal symbols, children who gesture will be communicating more content at earlier ages, and this in turn will increase language input at earlier ages.

Second, "a symbolic gesturing repertoire automatically increases the chance that parents will figure out what it is that the [child] wants to talk about" (Goodwyn et al., 2000, p. 99), and make that something the topic of conversation. This allows the child to direct cognitive resources towards language analysis rather than towards establishing joint attention, and increases the opportunities for language learning. The child who gestures will, in effect, set the topic for the ensuing exchange, and thus be more able to learn something new about language than if he or she had to first figure out what was being talked about.

Third, early use of gestures allows the toddler to experiment with symbols and discover the value of symbolic communication. These are areas of learning that generally do not occur until words are acquired. Indeed, our best understanding of the early one-word stage, with its persistently small vocabulary, is that this is the period during which children's first symbols—in this case, words—are slowly being decontextualized. Bates (1979) provides a good example of this process with observations about a child's use of the word *bam*. Initially, this noise merely accompanied the act of the knocking down a block tower, but soon *bam* became a word used as a request for someone else to knock the tower down, and finally as a comment on the blocks strewn about the floor. The really important fact about this process of decontextualization is that it stops being necessary. At a certain point in development, new words do not need to be laboriously decontextualized, but enter the repertoire as symbols from the outset. The child with gesture symbols can get to this point while using early signs, and thus will have a running start when word learning begins.

So Now What?

Many parents of normally developing children have been attracted by Goodwyn and Acredolo's work, seeing sign training as yet one more way to advance development. There is something vaguely disturbing about this parental drive for earlier and earlier achievement. First it was reading at age 3, now it's Mozart in the crib, and 11-month-olds talking like 15-month-olds. If you share my concern, you may wish to remind parents to pay attention to the entire set of results from Goodwyn et al. (2000). The language advantage seen in the second year largely disappears by age 3. There may be some lasting effect, but we don't yet have such evidence.

The reason I find this study valuable is not because I think we should accelerate normal development, but because these findings stand as strong proof that sign systems do not impede the learning of spoken language. This study also has caused me to think more deeply about the potentially positive effects of having a gesture symbol system before one can speak. There are good reasons to believe that early gestural symbols will increase input, facilitate joint attention, and demonstrate the power of symbolic communication. These consequences could be much more important for children with language learning problems than they are for normally developing children.

Using Sign in Intervention

The first study to look at the use of sign in language therapy with hearing children was conducted by Ellis Weismer and Hesketh (1993), with mixed outcomes. Sixteen young school children participated in a game in which they learned **nonce words** for location concepts (e.g., *beside* and *away from*). Half of the children had been diagnosed with SLI. For all participants, eventual comprehension was better for the terms that were presented with a gestural cue. In general, however, gestural cues did not facilitate the eventual production of the new words. Three children from the SLI group were exceptions to this rule, showing dramatic facilitation of word learning in the gesture condition.

Findings from a new study seem more promising. Robertson (2004) compared rates of vocabulary learning when new words were presented with versus without sign accompaniment. The children in the study were Late Talkers—2 to 2½ years of age, below the 5th percentile for size of expressive vocabulary, and showing good vocabulary comprehension. The study involved only two children, but each child received both sorts of treatment, with specific words assigned to each. The words were carefully selected to have developmentally early syllable shapes, sounds within the child's phonological system, and accessible meanings. The intervention was play based, with at least 10 models of each of 10 target words presented in each session. The study extended over 13 therapy sessions, encompassing 3 baseline sessions plus 10 treatment sessions. Each session utilized only one type of treatment and the two types were randomly ordered.

The results were clear and convincing. Both children ultimately produced more of the words that were presented with sign, and they learned them faster. These findings may be more positive than those in the earlier study because Robertson studied younger children at earlier stages of development, and used concepts for which the children did not already have words (i.e., her clinical population was more similar to the children in the Goodwyn et al. study).

Should we now start using this procedure? From the standpoint of standards for evidence-based practice, Robertson (2004) is a good example of a well-designed single subject study with controls (i.e., Level 5 from Essay 2). That's not very high on the evidence ladder, but it is appropriate for early investigations of a topic to be small in scale. As clinicians we can wait for this line of research to develop further, or we can use this treatment approach experimentally—aware that there is very little evidence but also that the existing evidence is, on balance, positive. This is certainly an area in which more research would be welcome.❖

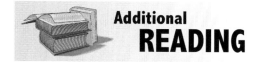

Additional
READING

Doherty, J. (1985). The effects of sign characteristics on sign acquisition and retention: An integrative review of the literature. *AAC: Augmentative and Alternative Communication, 1,* 108–121.

Questions for Discussion and
THOUGHT

1. This essay presents five reasons that signs or gesture symbols are easier to learn than speech and can actually facilitate oral language learning:

   - Signs can assist the recognition of spoken words.

   - Imitation of signs requires less transfer of information across sensory modalities.

   - Signs are communicative and thus engage conversational partners, increasing the amount of early language input.

   - Signs are symbols and allow the child to discover the nature and utility of symbolic representation prior to speaking.

   - Signs allow children to establish conversational topics for others to follow; which in turn frees the child from identifying the topic and allows more time for language analysis.

   Are some of these reasons more pertinent for children with autism (SLI, developmental delay, other disabilities) than others?

2. Which of the five facilitation mechanisms would also apply to the use of picture symbols, and which would not?

3. This essay focuses on children who are just beginning to talk. Can you extend the rationale for using total communication to school-age children as well? In what circumstances? And with which of the five facilitation mechanisms in mind?

Self-Guided Learning
ACTIVITIES

1. **Try with preschool children.** One interesting aspect of the Goodwyn et al. study is that they did not use ASL, Signed English, or any other formal sign system—they used gesture symbols that were highly iconic and ad hoc. The

researchers and the parents just made them up. If there is a child you are seeing who has a spoken/signed vocabulary under 25 words, try implementing such a program yourself. What advantages do you have by using self-created signs? What are the disadvantages? Does the nature of the child's problem affect your answers?

2. **Try with school-age children.** Review your caseload and select a child in third grade who has impoverished language and memory deficits. Now look at a recent lesson plan. Have you incorporated any visual learning supports? If not, find some way to do so (e.g., made-up symbols to accompany grammatical morphemes, Signed English).

30 Blackbirds and Fiddlers Three

When I was very young, my grandmother would sit with one leg crossed over the other, put me on her extended foot, and give me a ride. "Rida, rida ranka, Hasten heter Blanka, Vart ska vi rida?..." I can still hear the Swedish rhyme—the strange words that I knew meant something about horses, but mostly were about the pleasure of the game and our good times together.

The songs and poems that we now call nursery rhymes have been traced back as far as the thirteenth century. In those days, many of them were sung in taverns and had political or social significance. Centuries later, these texts no longer speak to us of the Plague, or of Jack Horner the steward to the Abbot of Glastonbury. "Jack and Jill," "Sing a Song of Sixpence," "Little Miss Muffet," and "Ring around the Rosie" are just nursery rhymes and, much to my surprise, I discover that I still know the words for many of them. Like "Rida Ranka," they are rhythmical, alliterative, and at times nonsensical. What does a pocket full of rye have to do with pie? And what are curds and whey, anyway? Some of the poems tell small stories, but even there we find repetition, special intonation, and words that rhyme.

In my childhood, and probably yours, nursery rhymes were all about fun with words, and about games with family and friends. But it turns out that they also have a role in promoting speech sound awareness and hence a link to literacy.

Nursery Rhymes and Reading

A number of researchers over the past two decades have looked at relationships between knowledge of nursery rhymes and performance on early reading tasks. In one frequently cited report, Bryant, Bradley, Maclean, and Crossland (1989) followed a group of 64 children over a three-year period as they entered school (CA 3;6–6;6). Even after controls for social background, IQ, and level of phonological development were put in place, knowledge of nursery rhymes at age 3 predicted success in reading and spelling three years later. This relationship is, of course, correlational and we know better than to assume too quickly that knowledge of these childhood rhymes is in itself the causal factor. But there is a larger research context that helps us interpret these findings—namely, the many studies that point to the importance of phonological awareness in the early stages of literacy.

Children who are consciously able to think about and manipulate the sounds of speech are apparently better prepared to learn phoneme-grapheme correspondences. In so far as nursery poems draw the child's attention to speech sounds and to rhythm and rhyme, they support the development of phonological awareness.

The Parent-Child Mother Goose Program

One outcome of this research on nursery rhymes is seen in the Parent-Child Mother Goose Program. All across Canada and Australia, groups of mothers with their preschool-age children meet weekly over a period of 10 weeks for an hour of rhymes, songs, and stories. The groups are sponsored by health units, schools, community centers, and other family resource agencies. For parents, the program provides opportunities to develop the good communication and observation skills that make parent-child interaction really enjoyable. For children, the program provides opportunities to develop new social skills as well as language and preliteracy skills.

Mother Goose groups are billed as preventative rather than as intervention or therapy, and this is an important distinction to keep in mind. Many of the participating families are economically disadvantaged and have limited education. I could find no outcome research, but I can imagine that 10 hours of parent education and general language stimulation could have a positive influence on children in such families—at least those who are typical learners. For children with language disorders, however, 10 hours of ordinary language stimulation is not likely to accelerate learning. More on that in a moment.

A study by Fernandez-Fein and Baker (1997) indicates the need for community programs such as Mother Goose. Four groups of children in prekindergarten classes (total N = 59) completed tasks in which they detected (or produced) rhyming words. The four groups were defined by economic circumstances (low income or middle income) and by ethnicity (European American or African American). The children were also asked to recite five common nursery rhymes, and the mothers were asked to complete a survey indicating their child's experiences with books, word play, and other early literacy activities.

Two findings from this study strike me as important. First, children from the low-income families spent less time playing word games and less time in book reading activities. Second, the best predictors of rhyming skills were maternal education (45 percent of variance), followed by nursery rhyme knowledge (12 percent), and ethnicity (5 percent). These findings suggest that children from economically disadvantaged homes may not have adequate access to the sorts of childhood texts that promote sound awareness.

Nursery Rhymes and SLI

We know that success in learning to read has at least two developmental roots: phonological awareness and general knowledge of language (see Essay 27). The first is particularly important in the child's early efforts to crack the code of written language; the second comes to the fore towards the end of grade 2 as children begin to read for meaning. Since they show limitations in both of these areas, children with specific language impairments are likely to have difficulties with reading, and many do.

Barb Fazio (1997b) decided to look further back in the developmental chain of events, at the knowledge and skill that might contribute to delays in phonological awareness. She compared 10 children with SLI to a group of control children matched for preschool classrooms. All participants were from low-income families. The experimental tasks explored memory for rote linguistic routines (counting, alphabet), sensitivity to rhyme, and knowledge of nursery rhymes. Children in both groups did well in reciting the alphabet, but there were strong group differences in the other areas. While their classmates could recite about 75 percent of five common nursery rhymes, the children with SLI could only recite about 35 percent, and they needed five times as many prompts to get even that far.

In a second task, Fazio (1997b) taught nursery rhymes to 16 low-income children in preschool programs, half of whom had been identified as SLI. As a pretest, each child attempted to recite eight common rhymes and participated in a rhyme detection task (choose the picture label that does not rhyme with the other two.) Following the pretest, all of the children received instruction on five of the rhymes that virtually no one had been able to recite. The lessons were presented to the entire classroom and included opportunities for the children to recite the rhymes in unison following the teacher's example. All five rhymes were practiced four days a week for six weeks. At the end of the training period, the assessment tasks were repeated by an examiner who knew neither the purpose of the assessment nor which children were in the SLI group.

At the outset of the instruction, the two groups of children had shown much the same recitation ability: Classmates 5 percent, SLI 2 percent. Following instruction, the children who were typical language learners could recite 68 percent of the rhymes, but the children with SLI only 20 percent of the rhymes. This group difference also carried over into the rhyme detection task. The children with SLI showed no improvement in identifying the word that didn't rhyme, but the classmates doubled their scores.

Fazio's final study (1997a) explored the efficacy of different teaching techniques. Once again she selected a group of low-income preschoolers with SLI. Two comparison groups were also formed: one comprised of classmates with similar age, gender, and race; the other comprised of younger children at the same language level, from similar social and economic backgrounds. All of the children were taught a novel rhyme in individual sessions over a four-week period. With some children, the therapist added a melody to the rhyme; with others, hand motions; with still others, both melody and motions; and with a final group, neither of these aids. The children with SLI needed two to three times more trials to learn the poem than children in *either* of the comparison groups. Two days later, children with SLI could remember only 50 percent of it, while children with normal language, regardless of age, could remember 80 percent. The one exception to this outcome was the children who were taught with hand motions. This group of SLI children came close to matching the performance of the normal learners.

Let the Fun Begin

Just barely knowing a nursery rhyme is not likely to have a literacy payoff. It is only when children are no longer struggling to remember the words that they can begin to reflect on and learn from the sound patterns in a nursery rhyme. Only then do nursery rhymes start being fun. How can we help children with language learning difficulties, from various diagnostic groups, achieve this level of mastery? One obvious way is to incorporate hand motions into the recitation of rhymes during the learning period. Fazio did not use ASL or other sign systems. Her gestures were more on the order of one per line to aid in recall (e.g., hands on the side of one's head with fingers pointing up to simulate mouse ears).

Here are some further ideas:

- **Ask parents to join the intervention process.** Choose a nursery rhyme for them to focus on, and have them practice the rhyme with their child. Nursery rhymes can be recited in cars, kitchens, bathtubs—places where more traditional therapies may be hard to incorporate.

- **Explore the possibility of culture-specific nursery rhymes with non-Western families** who may not have access to children's books in their home language or a cultural tradition of reading to children. They might be pleased to be able to focus on children's poems from their own culture, knowing that this activity will support later literacy learning. Perhaps you could learn one or more of these rhymes yourself.

- **Purchase nursery rhyme tapes** that you can loan out (e.g., the *Wee Sing Nursery Rhymes and Lullabies*).

- **Refresh your own memories or fill in some gaps** by visiting websites that provide the words to dozens of rhymes. Addresses tend to change at inconvenient times, but the following may help you find the useful sources:

  www-personal.umich.edu/~pfa/dreamhouse/nursery/rhymes.html
  This site has words for a huge list of rhymes.

  www.enchantedlearning.com/rhymes.html
  This site has activities and colorful learning materials for 29 rhymes.

  curry.edschool.virginia.edu/go/wil/rimes_and_rhymes.htm
  A-Rhyme-a-Week. This site has lesson plans and learning materials for 30 rhymes—in color and free to download.

A final thought for those of you who work with school-age children. Even though the content of this essay has focused on studies of preschoolers, nursery rhymes are definitely useful for primary-age children as well. Keep in mind that it is not the initial learning of the rhyme that has the payoff for phonological awareness, but the repeated recitation. If the children you see already know many of these rhymes, so much the better. You can use this knowledge to help them discover and consciously explore rhyme and alliteration. (See the advanced lessons on the Curry website.)❖

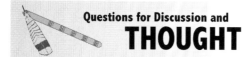

Questions for Discussion and THOUGHT

1. Fazio found that gestures aided the learning of rhymes, but melody did not. What other sorts of procedures or cues might help children learn and remember rhymes? Can you think of a way to visualize the rhyming elements? Or use scaffolding?

2. Would a child's language level influence his or her ability to learn nursery rhymes? In what way, and why?

3. When you select rhymes for a child to learn, which characteristics are important to consider?

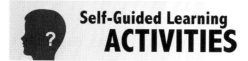

Self-Guided Learning ACTIVITIES

1. Choose a nursery rhyme that you do not already know. Ask a friend to tape-record the rhyme, reading with interesting intonation at a comfortable rate. Use this tape to learn the rhyme yourself. How many times do you need to hear it before you can repeat it all yourself? What sorts of errors do you make? What sorts of memory strategies do you use? Does it help to recite the rhyme along with the tape? After you finally succeed in reciting the rhyme, can you remember it five hours later? Two days later?

2. Repeat this exercise but instead of a nursery rhyme, learn the text from an early literacy book with predicable language patterns (e.g., those written by Joy Cowley; see note at the end of Essay 25). Try learning the story text with and without looking at the pictures in the book.

Facilitating Vocabulary Growth

T he average college graduate knows about 20,000 words, including roots with all their inflected and derived forms. This is an impressive achievement, and implies that somehow we have learned on the order of *three new words a day for 20 years* with a few days off for holidays. Rapid vocabulary growth begins during the preschool years. Once toddlers learn about 200 words, a vocabulary spurt occurs and they begin to actively seek word meanings, by pointing and asking, "What's that?" The rate of lexical learning slows in later adulthood, but vocabulary remains the one area of language that continues to develop throughout life. The Web will give you over 440,000 sites for the phrase *vocabulary size,* the *Reader's Digest* continues to offer "Thirty Ways to Improve Your Vocabulary," linguistic theory has dramatically reoriented towards the lexicon, and vocabulary test scores are regularly used as surrogates for IQ. So why, given the evident importance of vocabulary knowledge, have we heard so little about intervention in this domain?

Two answers to this question come to mind. First, I think we haven't understood the relationships between the lexicon and the grammar. We have focused on the grammar because combinatorial rules are the generative aspect of language knowledge, but in doing so we have ignored the symbiosis between words and sentence patterns. Syntactic information supports word learning, but once they are learned, words determine the grammatical options for each sentence. As SLPs we must include both the lexicon and the grammar in our intervention planning.

Second, I think that we have treated word learning too simplistically. We have been satisfied if a child is able to point to the correct picture on the PPVT or follow directions in the classroom. We have not paid attention to the breadth or depth of a child's knowledge of word meanings, to how words are organized, or how they are misused.

I lack experience in this domain as much as anyone else, but I am trying to learn. This section of the book includes three essays focused on lexical intervention—not because I understand it all, but because I am absolutely certain it is important.

31 The Skin of a Living Thought

A word is not a crystal, transparent and unchanged, it is the skin of a living thought and may vary greatly in color and content according to the circumstances and the time in which it is used.

—*Oliver Wendell Holmes, 1918*

Young children are remarkable word learners. Not only do they learn five words a day, they often do so from a small number of exemplars. Preschoolers can fast map an initial meaning onto a new sound string after only two to three hearings. These first meanings are quite restricted, however, especially in the case of verbs and adjectives. This restriction implies that word meanings must change and that there is a second, more protracted, stage of learning during which children elaborate their lexical representations until the meanings resemble those of the adult.

The literature on language intervention has seldom addressed lexical development. When it has, the focus has been largely on the first phase of word learning, when a new word enters the child's vocabulary. Given the key role of the lexicon in emergent syntax and effective communication, both of these biases are unfortunate. We need to be able to help children build their lexicon both by adding new words and by enriching the meanings of words they already know. Three recent studies provide guidance as we work towards these goals. But first, let's think about the fundamental differences between types of words.

Why Verbs May Be Hard to Learn

Although children are effective and rapid word learners, some words remain harder to learn than others. For example, toddlers learning English know more nouns than verbs. The first reason for this inequity concerns meaning. As argued by Gentner (1982), the *meanings of early verbs are more complex and variable than the meanings of early nouns*. Early nouns tend to refer to concrete objects in categories that are based largely on shape. Toddlers seem to discover this general principle and then use it to acquire hundreds of object names, often learning a new common noun after only one hearing. The meanings of early verbs, on the other hand, vary greatly from word to word and can refer to relationships, states, activities, changes of state, or causal events. Moreover, none of these meanings are neatly mapped to real world percepts. It is difficult to point to the referent of words such as *lose* or *show*.

Thinking About Child Language

To understand this difficulty, just imagine what a child might see when hearing the phrase "Feed the dog"—persons opening cans or bags, washing the dog dish or not, pouring dry pellets or spooning mash into variously shaped containers that are on the floor or not, a dog eating or not. As a second example, think about what a child might see when hearing the phrase "Put it away"—persons getting and carrying all sorts of objects, with all kinds of movements, to near and far away places, with a variety of final resting points. The permutations are many and there are few natural boundaries in these event streams. But even if there were tidy event segments with perceptual commonalities, the task of deducing meaning would not be simple. The way that verb meanings are lexically packaged is, in fact, not fully determined by the nature of the real world but depends greatly on the language being learned. English verbs of motion, for example, typically include *manner* (e.g., *run, skip, hop*) but not direction, while verbs in Romance languages include *direction* (e.g., *enter, exit*) but not manner. The first reason, then, that English-speaking children initially do not use many verbs is that the meaning of verbs is harder to deduce.

The second reason that English verbs are learned relatively late has to do with frequency of input. Cross-linguistic evidence has again been crucial in revealing this effect. Due to the nature of the language, children learning Mandarin do not hear as many nouns as children learning English, and it also seems that their vocabularies do not show the noun bias that is typical of English-speaking toddlers. Although there is some lingering debate surrounding these data, they seem to indicate that input frequency does help to shape the composition of the early lexicon. Other things being equal, children learn more of the words that they hear more often. For children learning English, this would predict early vocabularies that are noun-rich, and such is the case.

It turns out, however, that the relationship between input frequency and learning patterns is more complicated than the prior statement would suggest. Detailed frequency analyses of maternal speech in both Mandarin- and English-speaking homes (Sandhofer et al., 2000) reveal that there is a small subset of verbs that are actually heard at higher frequencies than any other words in maternal speech, but this fact does not necessarily lead to verb dominance. To the contrary, some of the verbs used most often by mothers in their speech to toddlers do not even appear in the child's early productive vocabulary (e.g., *remember, think, know*). Apparently, frequency of input is no guarantee of learning; we are reminded again that human development is usually determined by more than one factor.

Difficulties with Initial Stages of Lexical Learning

Windfuhr et al. (2002) report an experimental study of lexical learning by children with specific language impairments (SLI) and normally developing children (ND). There were 28 children in each group, ranging in age from 4;4 to 5;10 (SLI) and 2;4 to 3;7 (ND). Each child with SLI was carefully matched to a younger, normally developing child according to the number of regular verbs in their vocabulary and the likelihood of overgeneralization of verb inflections. Four new nouns and four new verbs were presented to each child during naturalistic play sessions. The new words were each spoken 10 times in each of four sessions, with suitable action and object accompaniments. Sessions occurred twice weekly, with the four verb sessions preceding the four noun sessions. Sessions were video-taped and transcribed, then all nonimitative uses of any of the new words were counted. The resulting data provide a measure of the children's success in initial word learning over a two-week period, for verbs versus nouns.

The most important findings from this study concerned verbs. Children with SLI learned fewer verbs than nouns, and fewer verbs than their language peers. The verb-learning trajectories for the two groups of children were very different, as well. The normally developing children attained their peak performance by session 2 and maintained this level of usage from that point onward. The children with SLI learned more slowly, using significantly fewer new verbs than the ND children during sessions 2 and 3. They essentially required three times the number of examples to approach the level of use seen in the ND group. This indicates a considerable degree of impairment if one keeps in mind that (1) the children in the ND group were more than two years younger than the SLI children, and (2) the groups had equivalent background knowledge of English verbs.

Facilitating New Verbs

The analyses of Gentner (1982) and Sandhofer et al. (2000) provide guidance for intervention in the area of lexical learning, especially verb learning. It is clear that we can affect learning patterns by increasing the frequency with which children hear specific words. This frequency effect is, however, constrained by a word's inherent difficulty. We can't merely provide repeated exposure to new words that are selected willy-nilly. Words differ in the complexity of their meanings, the degree to which they have perceptual correlates, and the availability of the concepts that they represent. These factors can guide our intervention plans for activities to facilitate verb learning. We've looked briefly at frequency; let's look now at the other three:

- **Meaning complexity.** Early verb meanings are more varied and more relational than early noun meanings. One widely used semantic taxonomy for
verbs and other relational words posits four major groups: activities/func-
tions, states, changes in state, and agents causing changes in state (Wells,
1985). Various syntactic and pragmatic cues can be used to decide which
words belong to which groups. For example, most verbs with agentive-
causal meanings can be used in the imperative *(Open the door immediately!)*,
while most verbs with stative meanings cannot be used in the imperative
*(*Hear the bird!)*. Table 31.1 lists 65 predicates (verbs, adjectives, other
relational terms) that children learn before the age of 4, grouped into these
major meaning categories (Dale & Fenson, 1996; Wells, 1985). Some words
can express two sorts of meaning depending upon context, and so are listed
twice. We can also group predicates according to the types of states that they
entail. For example, *buy, own, receive,* and *take* all entail some type of pos-
session, while *fix, broken, big, clean,* and *rough* all deal with physical states.
Although I know of no research on this point, we may be able to help children construct verb meanings by presenting together groups of verbs that
either share or contrast a specific feature of meaning. Sessions might focus,
for example, on verbs that refer to things changing their physical state (e.g.,
melt, grow, pop), or that refer to agents causing changes in physical states
(e.g., *break, fix, scratch*). Alternatively, we could present contrastive pairs
of verbs, one that refers to a state and one that refers to changes in that state
(e.g., *have/get, on/put, know/learn*). See Wells, 1985 for more examples.

- **Perceptual correlates.** Early verb meanings also do not have predictable perceptual correlates. A given verb typically refers to events or circumstances
that vary widely in their physical form. This makes it doubly important that
we not rely on pictured stimuli for verb learning. The defining elements of an
event are certainly not captured by the shape of a single exemplar (as is the
case for many nouns). The defining elements may not, in fact, be visible at all.
The verb *find,* for example, refers to a change in someone's knowledge/or
perceptual state. We may be able to picture the moment of discovery, but
how do we picture the earlier state of not knowing. Or, consider the verb
play. We can picture children surrounded by blocks, or swinging, or rolling

modeling clay, but how do we point to the common element of meaning in these activities? At the very least, we need to provide children real-time, three-dimensional experiences with events that illustrate the meaning of new verbs, and do so with multiple experiences and differing exemplars.

Examples of Verbs and Other Predicates,
Grouped by Type of Meaning*

Table 31.1

Activities/ Functions	States	Changes in State	Agents Causing Changes in State
26–30 Months**			
cry	big	find	build
blow	black	open	cook
chase	hard	break	draw
kiss	clean		clean
sing	cold		break
sleep	mine		make
swim	more		open
work	hear		call
	see		listen
30–48 Months**			
meow	a lot	lose	guess
laugh	messy	turn	sharpen
scream	one	catch cold	shine
pee	afraid	stay	squash
chew	angry	drip	call
bark	know	learn	count
hurry	belong	grow	decide
rest	dark	pop	teach
sneeze	different	melt	find out
	empty		fool

* At 42 months children's expressed meanings are distributed: 11% Activities/Functions, 45% States, 40% Changes in State or Agents Causing Changes in State (Dale & Fenson, 1996; Wells, 1985).
**Age at which at least 75% of children are reported to have spoken the word (Dale & Fenson, 1996; Wells, 1985).

- **Conceptual foundations.** Finally, children must have the conceptual tools necessary to construct the meanings of new verbs. Granted, language symbols do not map onto nonverbal concepts in a simple manner. Child language researchers have shown us that conceptual domains (e.g., space, family relationships, quantity) are organized in a language-specific fashion and, hence, that children must do more than merely associate preformed, universal meanings with new sound strings. This does not mean, however, that children's prelinguistic, nonverbal knowledge is irrelevant to verb learning; it means only that these early understandings must eventually be combined into the meaning bundles that are required by a given language. If children do not yet have the conceptual atoms that will make up the complex meanings of new verbs, they will be unable to interpret what they hear and see. This may be one of the reasons that mental state verbs such as *know* or *think* are not learned by toddlers even though the words occur frequently in maternal speech.

Difficulties with the Elaboration of Meaning

Helping children with the initial acquisition of a new word is just one aspect of lexically oriented therapy. School-age children with developmental language disorders frequently have problems with word-finding. Even after a word has entered their lexicon, they seem to have trouble recalling and using it appropriately. Karla McGregor at Northwestern University has been investigating word-finding difficulties for a decade now and one of her recent studies offers a new perspective on this problem. McGregor et al. (2002) used three tasks to explore the source of the naming errors made by school-age children with language disorders. In the first task, children named pictures of objects; in the second, they drew pictures of objects named by the examiner; and in the third task they gave definitions of object labels.

The children with language disorders made substantially more naming errors than did their age peers. The nature of the naming errors, however, was similar for the two groups. The most frequent error type was semantic substitution, the use of words with meanings that were related to the meaning of the target noun. For example, a child might say "music" instead of *stereo,* "saying hooray" instead of *cheering,* or "cutter" instead of *knife.* Neither of these findings was a surprise given earlier studies.

The new—and very important—finding from this study arose from the drawing task. For both groups of children, the items that had been misnamed were also the items which elicited the poorest drawings. These drawings were more likely to include irrelevant or inappropriate information than drawings for items that had been named correctly. For example, one child who correctly named a picture of a kite and later drew a perfectly recognizable picture of a kite, also said incorrectly that a pictured ax was a "hammer" and drew an unrecognizable blob when asked to draw an ax.

Data from the definition tasks corroborated this correlation between naming and quality of drawing. In the example given, the child explained that, among other things, "a kite is like you fly when wind," but said that an ax was "like a mow when you do your grass." Notice that this is not simply a case of not knowing the meaning of *ax*. The child had correctly represented some of the features of this object class (i.e., that axes are tools with cutting blades and are used outdoors). However, the meaning of the word was not fully understood and this sparse and/or inaccurate lexical representation was reflected in both naming and drawing.

McGregor's study was not designed with a language-match control group so it remains possible that the findings are merely a further reflection of the initial learning lag. It seems likely, though, that children with SLI continue to require still more time and more examples to achieve full understanding of a word's meaning once it enters the lexicon. Most importantly, the results from this study invite us to think about word finding in a new way. Instead of treating this problem strictly as a matter of memory recall, the data from the drawing suggest that we should look at word-finding errors as symptoms of incomplete or erroneous lexical representation. From this perspective, the problem is not one of finding, but of knowing.

Facilitating Later Stages of Vocabulary Development

Vocabulary knowledge changes and grows over time, not just because we learn more different words, but also because we learn more about each word. This is mastery learning in the lexical realm and it is similar to mastery learning in other areas of language. Word meanings must be thoroughly and robustly represented, or children will remain vulnerable to performance problems such as word finding. Unfortunately, the child language literature offers little general guidance to SLPs when it comes to the later stages of word learning. We know what mature lexical organization looks like, and we know how adults access words, but we don't yet understand the paths that lead to these competencies. Nevertheless, McGregor's work suggests some specific activities that should assist in vocabulary elaboration.

First, children can add features to word meanings by trying to compare and contrast members of a lexical family. What makes a lawn mower different from an ax? How many different garden tools (e.g., ways to move, things to eat, items to buy in a bakery) can we think of and what distinguishes them from each other? As you invent exercises of this sort, remember that most of the words should already be within the child's recognition vocabulary. That is, if you provided a relatively easy set of pictured alternatives (e.g., a cow, a scissor, a zinnia, and an ax), the child should be able to point to the ax when you name it. The goal of these exercises is elaboration, not initial learning.

Second, we can use drawing as a means of learning. Many children with language impairments learn best from visual information. I can imagine an activity in which the SLP and the child carefully observe and talk about new exemplars of nouns (*ax, doorway, lightning*) or verbs (*tip over, scowl, relay*) they have already met, then draw diagrams or pictures that highlight important features of meaning. The drawings needn't be expert. I recall a four-year-old who created a set of vocabulary cards with pictures that only he could recognize—but he did recognize them and delighted in using them to review his growing lexicon.❖

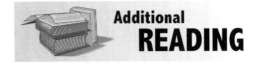

Additional
READING

Johnston, J., & Slobin, D. (1979). The development of locative expressions in English, Italian, Serbo-Croation, and Turkish. *Journal of Child Language, 6,* 529–545.

Wells, G. (1974). Learning to code experience through language. *Journal of Child Language, 1,* 243–269.

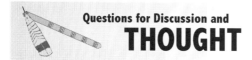

1. The four factors that determine the ease or difficulty of acquiring a verb appear to be: complexity of meaning, availability of perceptual correlates, availability of conceptual content, and input frequency. If so, what differences would we expect to see between normal learners and impaired learners? Why?

2. What is the most recent word you've added to your vocabulary? Why did you learn it so late? How would you rate your depth of knowledge for that word's meaning?

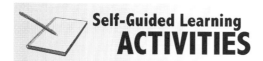

Self-Guided Learning
ACTIVITIES

The following eight verbs are normally learned by two- to three-year-olds: *do, drink, drop, go, pretend, push, run, think*. Make a chart and rate each verb 1, 2, or 3 for each of: meaning complexity, predictable perceptual correlates, conceptual availability, and input frequency. A rating of 1 would indicate the easier end of the continuum (i.e., meaning is simple, there are reliable perceptual correlates, the necessary concepts are available early, or the word is heard frequently).

When thinking about meaning complexity, think about factors such as whether the verb is causal, how many NPs it requires, or whether it implies an embedded complement sentence. Go with your instinct. It might be easiest to award the 1s and the 3s first, then give the remaining items, if any, a 2.

Add up the four ratings for each word to get a total score. On the basis of these totals, predict the order of acquisition for these words. Low scores should indicate words to be learned first. Now compare your predictions to the real-world facts, as listed at the end of Essay 33 on page 248. Did your predictions pan out? If not, why? Are there other factors we haven't included in the list, or is there some other explanation for the discrepancies?

32 And Inflections to Boot

I always imagined that when I booted my computer or used a boot disk, I was kicking life into the machine. It turns out, however, that the technoverb *to boot* doesn't mean *to apply one's boot to the side of,* but comes from the saying "to lift oneself up by one's bootstraps" (Weissman, 2001, p. 144). Taken literally, this metaphor doesn't make much sense. The scene it depicts would seem to be one of futility and stupidity, simultaneously pulling up and stepping down. Metaphorically, however, the phrase has come to mean *to help oneself without the aid of others; to use one's resources.* In the world of computers, the original bootstrap loader programs were very short programs that were just smart enough to read a slightly more complex program that then took control and read the operating system. These programs didn't know much, but what they knew was enough to get to the next stage. In the world of child language, bootstrapping likewise refers to the use of current, sometimes primitive, knowledge to learn something new.

Bootstrapping

The first appeal to bootstrapping in language acquisition came as theorists tried to explain how children figured out the meanings of early words and word combinations. They proposed that children use their nonverbal knowledge of objects and events to assign the most probable meanings to the language they hear, first to words and then to grammatical categories—a process that came to be known as *semantic bootstrapping* (e.g., Pinker, 1984). Since then, we've had *syntactic bootstrapping* (the use of sentence patterns to determine the meaning of new verbs), *prosodic bootstrapping* (the use of intonation contours to determine language segments), and more recently, *morphological bootstrapping* (Behrend et al., 1995).

Morphological Bootstrapping

Verb Meaning

To understand the process of morphological bootstrapping, we must first think about broad categories of verb meaning. One commonly used taxonomy comes from the work of Vendler (1957), who proposed that verbs can be divided into four groups according to meaning: states (e.g., *know, be in),* activities (e.g., *run around, play),* achievements (e.g., *arrive, win),* and accomplishments (e.g., *throw, open).*

These last two categories involve purposive actions directed towards an end result, and hence are referred to as telic from the Greek word *telos* (end, goal). Vendler's scheme is similar to the one used by Wells (1985) and described in Essay 31, except that Vendler focuses on the temporal contours of an event (e.g., whether or not it comes to an inherent end point) and the Wells scheme focuses on the participants (e.g., whether or not the event entails an agent).

These basic differences in verb meaning lead to predictable patterns of co-occurrence between English verb roots and inflections. Specifically, telic verbs are more likely to occur with the past tense *-ed* and activity verbs are more likely to occur with the progressive *-ing*. This is particularly true in the language addressed to, and used by, young children (Shirai & Anderson, 1995). We are more likely to talk about "eating your dinner" and "playing with Jimmy" than to remind a child that he "ate dinner" or "played ball." Similarly, we are more likely to comment when a child "broke the car" or "opened the purse" than to describe these events as they are happening, "You are breaking the car." Activities are not goal-oriented and they extend in time, thus inviting comment *while* they are underway. Telic events are goal-oriented and may be quite brief, thus inviting comment *after* the endpoint is reached. This frequent harmony between the inherent meanings of verbs and their companion inflections is what makes morphological bootstrapping possible. Young children can use their knowledge of inflectional meanings to categorize a new verb as being telic or atelic.

Inflectional Cues to Verb Meaning

Carr and Johnston (2001) report a study that shows how children use inflection to help them determine the meaning of a new verb. Ten 3-year-olds and eleven 4-year-olds participated in the experiment. The children watched a series of video segments, each showing a causal event (e.g., a rolling pin flattens a ball of clay). As the event unfolded, the researcher would introduce a new verb, inflected either with *-ed* or *-ing*, "Look. She biffed/is biffing." Then the child would see two additional events, one that preserved the action but changed the result (e.g., a rolling pin magically creates a gingerbread man) and one that preserved the result but changed the action (e.g., the end of a rolling pin presses down on the clay and flattens it). The child was told to select the event that was a second instance of *biff*. If the child chose the event that preserved the result, this indicated that he or she thought the meaning of the new verb was goal-oriented (e.g., cause-to-be-flat). If the child chose the event that preserved the action, this indicated that he or she thought the meaning of the new verb focused on the action rather than the result (e.g., roll-a-rolling-pin-over-clay).

There were two major findings from the experiment. First, the younger children clearly used the inflection on the novel verb to determine its meaning. If the verb was presented with the *-ed* inflection, they judged that its meaning included the result of the action; if the verb was presented with the *-ing* inflection, they judged that its meaning only included the action. The older children, in contrast, virtually always chose the result-oriented event regardless of the inflection, and judged all of the verbs to be telic.

These results suggest that during one phase of development, children use morphological cues to help determine the initial meanings of verbs. From prior language input and their own language use, children have discovered the common patterns of co-occurrence between root and inflection, and this knowledge guides their learning. Morphological bootstrapping is certainly not the only route to meaning. Sentence patterns, discourse context, analysis of prior lexical entries, and event interpretation also shape semantics, but grammatical inflection is nevertheless a potent cue.

What about the older children? Carr and Johnston (2001) speculate that as children begin to talk more about events removed from the here and now, and also engage in more storytelling, they learn that inflection is not a completely reliable cue to verb meaning. Activity verbs can, after all, occur in the past tense, particularly in narrative. This realization, coupled with the fact that the final screen of the video segment always showed a resulting state, may explain why older children preferred telic meanings.

Broken Bootstraps or Bare Feet?

In a second study, Carr and Johnston (2001) asked four-year-olds with specific language impairments to do the experimental task. These children had significant language delays, and may have had more difficulty with grammatical morphemes than with other aspects of the system (Johnston, 1988). All of them, however, were using *-ed* and *-ing* in spontaneous speech. Despite this prior knowledge, the children with SLI showed no evidence of morphological bootstrapping and no clear pattern of event preference.

We have long known that grammatical morphology is less well developed than sentence patterns or the lexicon in the speech of many children with SLI. This is one of the factors that make their complex sentences difficult to understand. The

Carr and Johnston (2001) data suggest another consequence of morphological deficits. Primary-age children with serious language impairments may be unable to use morphology as a cue to the meaning of new verbs. They may fail to notice the inflection, or may lack the capacity needed to operate on such cues. Whatever the nature of the deficit, this particular bootstrap seems to be broken.

Does this mean that children with language impairments must tackle verb meaning without the advantages of morphological bootstrapping? Probably, but morphology is not the only possible cue. As they make their initial estimates of meaning, children can also draw on information from the lexicon, the discourse context, the speaker's attentional focus, the nature of the event, and the overall sentence pattern. Every verb that is learned implies the successful use of one or more types of cue. Research on these topics is sparse, but a few recent studies have shown how even children with SLI use sentence patterns to determine verb meaning (e.g., O'Hara & Johnston, 1997). There is no a priori reason to imagine that they cannot use the other sorts of information as well.

Teaching New Verbs

Children with SLI, like all language learners, use their prior knowledge of language and the world to lift themselves up to new knowledge states. They may not be able to use morphological bootstrapping, but this does not mean they must approach language with no boots at all. The challenge for interventionists is to make sure that all possible cues to meaning are in fact present, and that in our effort to structure the learning environment we haven't removed the very information that is needed. The literature on early lexical development suggests a number of ways we can help children learn new verbs.

- **Use real contexts.** Introduce new verbs as labels for real-time, three-dimensional events, rather than represent them with pictures.

- **Provide an informative range of referents.** Use the new verb in more than one event context, varying the event parameters so children can decide whether, for example, the verb is action oriented or goal oriented.

- **Let syntax help.** Introduce new verbs in simple, but prototypical sentence patterns that themselves convey basic meanings (e.g., NVN with a direct object when the verb is causal).

- **Link to familiar verbs of the same type.** Use the new verb in activities that highlight the similarities in meaning between verbs of a given type, such as telling dolls to perform a series of activities that are all noncausal (e.g., *swim, walk, sneeze, hop, play*) rather than a series that mixes causal and noncausal event types (e.g., *run, break, make, swim*).

Consistent attention to these features of the learning environment should optimize the child's efforts to acquire new verbs.❖

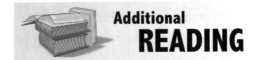

Additional
READING

Shirai, Y., & Anderson, R. (1995). The acquisition of tense aspect morphology. *Language, 71,* 743–762.

Naigles, L., & Hoff-Ginsberg, E. (1995). Input to verb learning: Evidence for the plausibility of syntactic bootstrapping. *Developmental Psychology, 31,* 827–837.

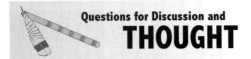

Questions for Discussion and
THOUGHT

1. Linguists now emphasize the centrality of verbs in the organization of virtually all language knowledge. Review your caseloads and learning goals. Is vocabulary a high priority, especially the learning of new verbs? If not, what are some of the reasons—maybe good, maybe poor—that you aren't spending more time in that domain? Is there any action plan implicit in your answers?

2. Go around the circle, each person describing an activity that she or he has recently used to facilitate verb learning. For each one, look back at the guidelines at the end of the essay and discuss how or if the activity could be improved.

3. Do you know of any research that would help us decide how many related words to introduce at one time? What does your own experience as an L2 learner suggest?

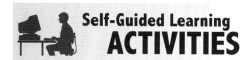 **Self-Guided Learning**
ACTIVITIES

1. **Try with preschool children.** Go to the norms for the CDI (www.sci.sdsu.edu/cdi). Ask to see the data for action words at 30 months, in order of frequency. This will give you a list of about 100 verbs that are produced by almost all normally developing children at age 30 months. Print out the list. For each verb, decide which type of meaning it expresses: telic or atelic (or don't know). Try using this list to guide you as to which inflection to use as you introduce that verb.

2. **Try with school-age children.** Take a language sample that is already transcribed, and make a list of all the verbs that the child uses, along with their tense form (i.e., progressive *-ing* or past-tense *-ed* and irregulars. (If you have access to the SALT program, this is easily done by asking for a list of all the bound morphemes along with the word roots on which they appear. Otherwise you could use your word processor to find the tense forms, or just scan for verbs by eye). Is there an even distribution of tense forms for telic and atelic verbs? Does the same verb get used with both inflections, or just one?

33 An Anatomy of Verb Learning

Several years ago, undergraduates at the University of Pennsylvania learned the hard way why early vocabularies are full of nouns, not verbs. Gillette et al. (1999) asked them to watch video-taped segments of mothers playing with toddlers. In each edited segment there were six instances of a mother using a given verb. The students were to watch the set of interactions and guess which verb was being used. There was no audio on the tapes, but to make the task easier, the experimenters included only the verbs that were most frequently used in maternal speech, and they inserted a beep just at the moment that the verb was being used. How well do you think the university students did?

There would be many reasons to expect success: the students had the necessary concepts, they were seeing six instances of the same verb right in a row, and they actually knew the word already. Moreover, this is pretty much what young children do all the time—observe the situation, listen to the noises, and guess what they mean. If children can do it, why should it be hard for college students? In fact, the students failed this task miserably, guessing correctly on only 8 percent of the items. This finding raised important questions about what young children are doing when they learn new words. In subsequent tasks the researchers varied the sources of information that were available to the students, in effect dissecting the process of learning. The resulting picture of verb learning is fascinating and very applicable to intervention practice.

Inside Verb Learning

Gillette et al. (1999) identify three quite different types of information that can be used to determine the meaning of a new verb: the nonverbal context, the key nouns in the sentence, and the syntactic frames in which those nouns appear. Let's think about each in turn.

Nonverbal Context and Imagability of Referent

The nonverbal context can be useful in learning the meaning of certain verbs, but it also presents challenges. Events and relationships do not come in neatly bounded packages the way that objects do; children must decide where one event ends and the next one begins. Also, events or relationships of a given kind do not physically resemble each other in the same way that objects do. Children must go beyond form and consider more abstract similarities. Think, for example, about the class of objects called *fish* and the class of events called *sell*. *Fish* have similar shapes and patterns of movement, and they are only found in water, in the market, or on one's plate. *Sell,* on the other hand, refers to a range of events that have virtually no physical similarity—the man in the used car lot, the real-estate weekly, the beer vender in the sports arena, and so forth. It would be difficult for children to find the similarity between these instances from perceptual data alone.

Pursuing this idea, Gillette et al. (1999) asked the students to rank all the nouns and verbs in the video segments according to the ease with which they evoked a mental image, or, in other words, according to their association with specific perceptions. Imagability turned out to be a better predictor of whether a word would be known by a 20-month-old than syntactic class was. The researchers concluded that it isn't so much that early vocabularies are filled with nouns, but that they are filled with words referring to objects or events that have strong perceptual correlates—most of which happen to be nouns.

Co-occurring Nouns

A second source of information about the meaning of a new verb is the set of nouns with which it co-occurs. In the simple speech addressed to toddlers, the nouns in a sentence are likely to refer to the different things (e.g., objects, ideas, places, persons) that are inherently entailed in the meaning of the verb. The number and nature of these things can indicate much about this meaning. As an example, consider the verbs *break* versus *give*. *Break* refers to events that inherently involve two things: the *break-er* and the *brok-en*. *Give,* on the other hand, refers to events that inherently involve three things: the *giv-er, giv-en,* and *giv-ee*. Notice too that the set of things that will be mentioned along with *break* or *give* will always include one that is animate and one that is inanimate, while the thing mentioned with the verb *vibrate* should always be inanimate. Even with these simple examples you can begin to see how much information about the meaning of a new verb can be inferred from the nouns in the sentence. If you knew that a new verb entailed two things, one of which was animate, you could immediately narrow your initial guesses about meaning. When the Penn students were given only the sets of nouns that co-occur with a verb, arranged alphabetically, they were able to guess the verb in 17 percent of the items, even without the video. When the video was added to the noun clusters giving them access to the event context, they could identify 29 percent of the verbs!

Thinking About Child Language

Syntactic Frames

A third source of information about the meaning of a new verb is its syntactic frame. The phrase-structure patterns in which a verb occurs strongly predicts whether it refers to causal relations (transitive N + V + N), movement and transfer events (N + V + PP), physical states (BE + Adj), and so forth. To test the value of syntactic information, Gillette et al. (1999) gave the Penn students written transcripts of all the various instances of each verb, but replaced all the content words with nonsense words. For the verb *call*, for example, students saw:

"Why don't ver GORP telfa?" (Why don't you call Daddy?)

"Can ver GORP litch on the fulgar?" (Can you call Mum on the phone?)

"Mek gonna GORP litch," (I'm gonna call Daddy.)

"GORP litch." (Call me.)

It turned out that the set of frames for a given verb carried surprisingly rich information about its meaning. Even without the video, this syntactic information led to 52 percent success in identifying verbs! When real nouns were added back in, the success rate rose to 75 percent. And finally, when the students could use all three sources of information—the video, the real nouns that co-occured with the verb, and the syntactic frames—they identified an impressive 90 percent of the verbs in the mothers' speech.

The researchers point out that in the real world, there are also social, prosodic, and morphological cues to verb meaning. They also acknowledge that toddlers, unlike college students, may not always have the necessary conceptual resources. Even bearing these caveats in mind, the Gillette et al. (1999) study provides a fascinating analysis of verb learning. Table 33.1 shows the numbers.

I find it interesting that, taken one at a time, the linguistic sources of information are more useful than the nonlinguistic, and that syntactic information is the most useful of all. This may be part of the explanation for the rapid increase in verb vocabulary that accompanies early word combinations. What Gillette and colleagues are proposing here is a linked series of bootstrapping dependencies. Children use their knowledge of real-world objects to learn a set of nouns. Patterns of co-occurring nouns then give them cues to the nature of English clausal structure. Finally, armed with new, clause-level syntax, children can rapidly learn new verbs.

Table 33.1   **Cue Value of Different Information Sources**

Source	Value
Nonverbal context	7.7%
Co-occurring nouns	16.5%
Nonverbal context *and* co-occurring nouns	29.0%
Syntactic frame	51.7%
Syntactic frame *and* co-occurring nouns	75.4%
Syntactic frame *and* co-occurring nouns *and* nonverbal context	90.4%

Source: Gillette et al. (1999)

Children with Language Learning Difficulties

We know from Carr and Johnston (2001) that children with SLI may fail to use morphological cues to verb meaning (see Essay 31). But what about other bootstrapping opportunities? I know of no research on the ability of poor language learners to use only noun-cluster or only nonverbal information to infer meaning. However, there have been several studies in which children with SLI have been asked to use *syntactic bootstrapping* to ascertain the meaning of a new verb. In these studies, nonce verbs are presented in otherwise grammatical English sentences and the child is supposed to act out the meaning of the sentences with small toys. This would be similar to the Gillette et al. (1999) condition which presented both the co-occuring nouns and the clause structure—a condition that led to success on 75 percent of the verbs.

O'Hara and Johnston (1997) presented one such syntactic bootstrapping task to six children with SLI (age 7;9) and six children with normally developing language (age 6;2) who were matched by sentence comprehension scores on the

TOLD. There were 18 items, evenly divided among three types of sentences: transitive (*The woman soogs the bunny*); transitive locative (*The bear gebs the boy to the woman*); and transitive with conjoined object NPs (*The bunny bims the farmer and the cow*). At first it seemed as though the children with SLI were very limited in their ability to use linguistic cues to infer verb meaning. Across sentence types, they correctly acted out only 43 percent of the sentences while their younger language-peers correctly acted out 87 percent of the sentences.

However, when we looked at the items on which the SLI children had made errors, we noticed something important. It was not always the verb that was the problem. In many cases, the children had selected the wrong toys or assigned the various players to the wrong roles, but had acted out the right sort of verb. In fact, when we scored *just* the verbs, the children with SLI were successful 70 percent of the time. While still lower than the score of the children with normally developing language, this score indicated that the children with SLI could use syntactic bootstrapping to infer the meaning of a new verb. Limitations in working memory, inefficiencies in syntactic analysis, or some combination of the two apparently led to sentence comprehension errors, but the children's capacity for learning verb meanings from syntactic information was very real.

Helping Children Learn Verbs

One reason that Gillette et al. (1999) caught my attention is that it shows so clearly the separate sources of information that contribute to vocabulary learning, and the additive nature of these contributions. If the pool of undergraduates had been larger, or the granting agency more generous, the researchers might have added other sources to their model, such as morphology or speaker intentionality. But the three sources they chose made the point quite nicely and also allowed them to demonstrate the developmental priorities inherent in these sources of information. We can rephrase their findings as principles for language therapy.

Principle 1. Language learners are more successful in figuring out the meaning of new words when they have more different kinds of information to draw on. We should maximize the diversity and number of cues.

Principle 2. Different sorts of cues to word meaning are available and needed at different stages of language development. We should set learning goals that are in accord with the possible sources of information.

This second principle is particularly important for children at the one- and two-word stage. Given the importance of verbs in language representation, it is tempting to set verbs as the goals for early learning. The Gillette et al. (1999) study indicates, however, that verbs will be much easier to learn *after* the child has acquired basic clause patterns (e.g., N + V, N + V+ PP, N + V + N, N + BE + Adj). These patterns could be acquired by teaching only a small set of high frequency verbs such as *put, go, want*, and *be*.

Once the basic clause patterns are available, new verbs can be systematically presented so as to contrast their possible frames. For example, think about the two verbs *eat* and *smile*. Both involve the mouth, both occur in social settings, and both could conceivably be uttered while sitting with one's family at the table. Nonverbal cues to meaning could thus be quite confusing. However, while both of these verbs can occur in intransitive frames (i.e., N + V), only *eat* can also occur in a transitive frame (i.e., N + V + N). And, while both can occur with prepositional complements, the N in the prepositional phrase associated with *eat* is a location but the N in the prepositional phrase associated with *smile* is likely to be a person or object. These facts suggest that we should use a range of sentences such as: "Big Bird is eating his dinner. There. He's eating. He's eating more. He's eating in the kitchen. Ah, he's smiling. Look. Now Kermit is smiling. He's smiling at Big Bird." The argument here is not that we need to teach the child the contexts in which the verb can occur, but that syntax can help the child to figure out verb meanings. By presenting new verbs in a generous sampling of the syntactic frames in which they are allowed, we can give the child basic information about verb semantics.

This is not to say that nonverbal cues have no value. To the contrary. Syntactic cues alone might lead the child to assign meanings such as *go* and *drive* to the new verbs *eat* and *smile*. It is important that these verbs are being used at the dinner table, as food is being eaten. But note the third principle that was demonstrated in the Gillette et al. (1999) data:

Principle 3. Nonverbal information is twice as valuable when it accompanies rich linguistic cues than when it is presented alone.

Finally, although some researchers would disagree with me, I believe that the principles outlined above apply to children with language learning difficulties just as much as they apply to normally developing children. Since they stem from the inherent nature of language and language learning, they cannot be compromised. As is suggested by O'Hara and Johnston (1997), verb learning may sometimes be hidden by performance difficulties. But if we provide children, even poor language learners, with the full complement of nonverbal and linguistic cues to meaning, they should be able to build an initial lexical entry that is heading in the right direction.❖

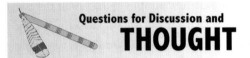

Questions for Discussion and
THOUGHT

1. Is there anything inherently different about intervention in vocabulary learning that sets it apart from work on syntax or morphology? If any of these differences create challenges for therapy planning, what could be done to minimize them?

2. If syntactic cues provide valuable cues to the meaning of new words, why do we so often use truncated, telegraphic speech to children with learning disorders? What are the assumptions of this practice? Do you know of pertinent evidence?

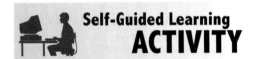

Self-Guided Learning
ACTIVITY

Go the website of the MacArthur-Bates Communicative Development Inventory (www.sci.sdsu.edu/cdi). Look for the normative data and write down the 25 verbs that appear to be learned at the earliest ages. After each verb on the list, indicate the syntactic patterns it will fit into. You could start with the following patterns: (1) N + V, (2) N + V + N, (3) N + V + PrepPhrase, (4) N + V + N + PrepPhrase, (5) N + V + Embedded Sentence. Do you see any similarities in the meaning of the verbs that fit into the same clusters of sentence patterns?

Answers to activity for Essay 31: The order of acquisition is as follows: (1) *go;* (2) *drink;* (3) *do, run* [tied for 3.5]; (5) *push;* (6) *drop;* (7) *think;* and (8) *pretend.* Order is taken from the month at which the word is produced by at least 50% of the children in the CDI database.

Responding to Diversity

When I set off back to school, some 35 years ago now, my goal was to figure out what language intervention was and why it worked. My answer was "Fit, Focus, and Functionality" (Essay 21)—a theory of intervention that could be applied to all children, regardless of age, language level, or diagnosis. Some of my colleagues are bothered by the universality of this claim. Certainly it runs counter to much of the textbook literature where we find lengthy comparisons of the syntactic approach versus the pragmatic approach, or elicited imitation versus modeling techniques. Given my long-term commitment to generic intervention, it may surprise you to see that the next section of this book includes five essays on diversity that are chock full of suggestions about how our interventions can be, and must be, individualized.

The tension between the universal and the particular in this case is more apparent than real, and can be resolved in two complementary ways. First, the notion of systematic differences is an important middle ground between the extremes of the generic and the individual. In each child we see a particular combination of learning style, interests, culture, intellectual and emotional strengths, social experience, developmental level, and much more. But it is the combination that is unique. Considered individually, these various aspects of personhood are shared and can be studied and understood in a general fashion. In the essays to follow, you will find some of what it means to say that Raul is a bilingual Hispanic boy who is a Gestalt language learner at Level 2. Those facts, even doubled or tripled, wouldn't begin to capture the child we know, his love of learning, or what makes him smile, but they can help us select from our therapy options the ones that are most likely to fit.

A second resolution to the apparent conflict between generic therapy and the need to individualize lies in the level of analysis. "Fit, Focus, and Functionality" (FFF) concerns abstract principles, not content, procedures, or activities. Even if you adopt FFF as a planning and evaluating framework, you still will need to make many decisions about the specific language pattern that a given child needs, about the types of discourse engineering you will use, and about the activities that will make the learning experience both motivating and fun. Principles can be generic, but content, procedures, and activities require us to think about diversity.

34 Everybody's Different

Here's a question for you. Which principles or facts about normal language acquisition are important to keep in mind when planning intervention? When my students answer this question, they may list developmental stages, environmental input, genetic predispositions, perhaps even universal grammar or prosodic bootstrapping. But always, someone will say that it is important to remember that every child is different.

However true it may be, I find this idea challenging. The notion that everyone is different is actually not a very useful starting place for thinking about intervention. Taken to the extreme, the idea that everyone is different would leave us totally without guidelines for practice. Educational planning requires us to generalize our experiences from one child to another on the assumption that they are in some ways the same, not different. Why, then, does this idea always emerge? Probably out of some desire to avoid overly general stereotyping, but also, I suspect, out of our own strong sense of personal identity. Logically, I may argue for looking only at general principles, but down deep I do understand the desire to be known as one of a kind. The challenge is to find a balance between the utility of the general and our respect for the individual.

One approach to balancing these two perspectives is to think systematically about individual differences, to look for *patterns* of behavior and learning that distinguish one *group* of children from another. In this way, SLPs can work with general principles while at the same time acknowledging that not every child is the same. A recent study by Michigan researchers shows the benefits of this approach.

Beyond the Reading Wars

A research team led by Carol Connor is trying to broker an end to the reading wars by showing that both whole language and phonics are needed, and also that they need to be flexibly combined in different mixes (Connor et al., 2004). Briefly, the project followed 108 children in 42 first-grade classrooms in a large midwestern American city. Children were assessed in a number of areas, including reading and language. In the initial testing sessions, the PPVT was used to measure vocabulary and the Reading Recognition subtest of the PIAT was used to measure letter identification, letter-sound correspondences, and single word recognition (a cluster of reading skills hereafter called *decoding*). The researchers also made extensive observations in the classroom at three points during the year, recording the amount of time spent on specific types of instructional activity.

The scheme used by Connor et al. (2004) for categorizing these activities is interesting and deserves some attention. There were two main dimensions in the coding scheme: (1) explicit versus implicit, and (2) teacher managed versus child managed. *Explicit* activities were those that addressed a specific skill directly and in a highly focused manner, (e.g., teaching phonological awareness or letter names). *Implicit* activities were those that might indirectly lead to improvement in a skill. For example, reading a text for meaning might lead a child to discover some new aspect of decoding, but that would not be the focus of the activity. *Management* of an instructional activity referred to exactly that (i.e., the person who directed the activity in the moment). Note that this was not necessarily the person who created the activity. A teacher might create a worksheet, but if the child then took it and worked on it independently, this activity would be considered child managed. A third dimension of instruction ultimately emerged from the longitudinal observations, and this was the degree to which the classroom activities changed in character over the course of the year.

The Road to Success in Decoding

For this particular report, the researchers investigated the relationships between improvement in decoding scores over the course of the year and the type of instruction the children received. They found strong predictive relationships, *but only if they first considered both vocabulary and decoding skills at the beginning of the year*. The results can be summarized as follows. Children who entered first grade with vocabulary and decoding skills below the 25th percentile made more improvement in decoding abilities when there was relatively more Teacher-Managed Explicit (TME) instruction in this aspect of reading, and less time spent in Child-Managed Implicit (CMI) instructional activity (e.g., silent reading). Interestingly though, the greatest growth for these children was seen when this relatively small amount of CMI activity increased steeply over the course of the year. The reported differences were not trivial. Two children starting out with the same scores, but in optimal versus nonoptimal classrooms, could vary in their decoding scores by as much as two grade equivalents by the end of the school year!

Similar stories emerged for the three other groups of children who were identified in this project. Children with low decoding scores but high vocabulary scores (90th percentile) did best when they received relatively high amounts of both kinds of instruction and these high levels were maintained throughout the year. Children who entered first grade with high decoding skills but poor vocabulary did best when the classroom began with low levels of Child-Managed Implicit instruction (remember, this often consisted of silent reading) but strongly increased these levels over the year. For them, the amount of TME in decoding skills was essentially irrelevant. Individual children within either of these two groups could vary as much as one and a half grade equivalents by the end of the year depending on which sort of instruction they had received. And finally, children who entered first grade at the 90th percentile in both domains, not surprisingly, continued to do well regardless of what happened in the classroom.

General Lessons on Teaching and Learning

Like you, I suspect, I found the description of the teaching activities in this report rather frustrating. The phrases *Teacher-Managed Explicit instruction* or *Child-Managed Implicit instruction* don't seem to capture the essence of rhyming games or silent reading. The full implications of this study do not, however, derive from these descriptions. I see four broader lessons here that we can all learn from, even those of us who never enter a primary classroom.

- **No one-size fits all.** First, notice that there was no one best type of reading instruction! What was best for a child depended on the learning resources that the child brought into the classroom (i.e., what the child already knew and could do). Development is always interactive between the environment (that's us) and the child.

- **Change happens.** Second, notice that especially for the children with low vocabulary scores, the way that the instruction changed over the year was important. How easy it is for us to forget that each time a child learns something new, we have a new child with new learning capabilities. The activity that didn't work last winter may now be perfect.

- **Determining factors interact.** Third, in order to find these predictive relationships, the researchers had to characterize the child in a complex fashion. Initially they just looked at *either* vocabulary or decoding scores and found no useful trends. It was only when they considered both scores at once that their data made sense. In the world of spoken language, we may need to do the same. Children who initially seem to have the same problem may be behaving similarly for quite different reasons. Imagine, for example, two children at the three-word stage with poor use of grammatical morphology. It may look at first as though these children would profit from the same intervention approach. However, what if one of the children has a normal range vocabulary score and the other one shows vocabulary delays? We know from the literature on normal child language that morphosyntactic development requires a robust vocabulary as well as auditory perceptual analysis. Taking the cue from Connor et al. (2004) we may want to consider very different intervention approaches for these two children, one concentrating on vocabulary growth, the other on perceptual salience. But we can only make this and other such decisions by considering a whole range of facts about the child, not just the single low score in morphology.

- **Best practice is specific to the goal.** Finally, the patterns of effective instruction very much depended on the learning goals. Although my summary doesn't emphasize this, the authors are very clear that these instructional predictions apply only to progress in decoding skills, not reading comprehension. They intend to address this aspect of reading in a separate study.

Individual Differences in Language Learning and Language Intervention

Connor et al. (2004) demonstrate the importance of individualizing our language interventions. In order to do so, we need to consider the ways that language learners can be systematically different. Gender and culture differences are important, and other essays in this section address those topics. The literature on normal language development suggests at least one further dimension of difference, namely, the early use of unanalyzed phrases. Some children seem to focus on noun labels for object classes as their entrance point to the language system, while other children begin with many phrase-like chunks of language that are used in social routines such as "That's mine," "I do it," or "What's that?"

I know of no studies that look systematically at the intervention strategies that best serve the Analytic versus the Gestalt learner, but a book by Ann Peters (1973), *The Units of Language Acquisition*, has excellent ideas for helping children move from phrase knowledge to word knowledge. The book is out of print, but Ann has made it available to new readers by publishing it on the Web (www.ling.hawaii. edu/faculty/ann).

Intervention Adapted to Differences

Language intervention research has not yet grappled seriously with the implications of systematic individual difference. We have focused on program variables and on the development and general efficacy of intervention strategies, but have tended not to include child variables in the equation. We attend to the child's language level when selecting learning goals, but less so when making decisions about our basic approach. But even if we had a definitive list of dimensions such as Gestalt/Analytic and could thoroughly describe the child, we would not have all of the information we need because we don't yet know which approaches fit which sorts of children. There is every reason to believe that, just as in reading instruction, the best language intervention for a given child will depend on systematic facts about that child's current knowledge and learning style—but which facts? Linked to which program variables?

Researchers have sometimes invoked individual differences as a post hoc explanation for disparate findings, and we have a growing body of studies that compare two approaches to intervention with the same group of children. What we lack is the complementary body of research that charts the outcomes for a single approach used with different groups of children. Over the last 25 years there seems to have been only one or two such studies. The clearest set of findings is found in Friedman and Friedman (1980). This team used a programmed imitative approach with some children and an interactive focused-stimulation approach with others. Initially the two approaches seemed to be equally effective, but when child variables were factored into the analysis, a different conclusion emerged. Children with high IQ, advanced syntax levels, and intact visual motor integration showed more syntactic improvement with the interactive approach, while children with lower initial scores on these measures improved more with the programmed approach.

What we need now are more studies of this sort with a current set of predictive variables and therapy approaches. Larry Leonard recently came to the same conclusion following his comprehensive review of the intervention literature: "we have not reached a point of knowing which approaches are the most effective for teaching particular targets...or which children will benefit most from particular treatment approaches" (Leonard, 1998, p. 204).

A welcome addition to the therapy literature will soon be available as results from the clinical trials investigating the outcomes of the Fast ForWord® program are published (Gillam, 2005). This large sample study compares the gains made by 6- to 8-year-olds after 30 days of intensive intervention in one of four modes: computer-based language games with acoustically altered speech; computer-based language games with ordinary speech; computer-based games in math and social studies; and traditional interaction with a therapist using narrative-based activities. Findings from this project will not only tell us whether these programs work, but also will help to identify the sorts of children for whom they work best. Preliminary reports again indicate that the four therapy approaches had relatively similar outcomes, at least in the short term, until you factored in the child's initial language level and socioeconomic level. With this subdivision, the various approaches led to different outcomes for different groups of children.

Connor et al. (2004) present classroom teachers with a gigantic challenge: how to meet the learning needs of a diverse group of children in a single classroom. SLPs are more fortunate in that we often have the luxury of working with individual children or small groups that we compose ourselves. What we need now is research that will move us beyond "everybody's different" to an understanding of the systematic differences among learners that can help us optimize our intervention.❖

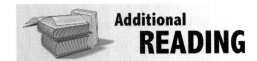 **Additional**
READING

Peters, A. (1973). *The units of language acquisition*. Cambridge, UK: Cambridge University Press.

Wetherby, A., & Prizant, B. (2005). Enhancing language and communication development in autism spectrum disorders: Assessment and intervention guidelines. In D. Zager (Ed.), *Autism spectrum disorders: Identification, education, and treatment* (3rd ed., pp. 327–365). Mahwah, NJ: Erlbaum.

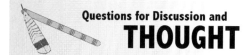

Questions for Discussion and
THOUGHT

1. Make a list of the dimensions of individual difference that you think need to be considered when planning therapy. When you have an opportunity, give your list to your friendly university researcher. We value this sort of input from our clinical colleagues.

2. Besides individuality, what normal language facts and principles do you think are important for SLPs to keep in mind? Give concrete examples of how each of them would influence practice.

3. What aspects of language therapy do not recreate the normal circumstances of learning? What do you do that makes the child's learning opportunities extraordinary and, hence, therapeutic? Can you explain why?

4. What would be the effects on your initial assessment and ratings of progress if a child on your caseload were a Gestalt learner?

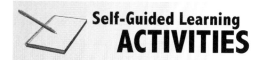

Self-Guided Learning
ACTIVITIES

1. **Try with preschool children.** Review your caseload and choose one or two children who are just beginning to combine words. This developmental level is the point at which it is important to determine whether a child is relying on unanalyzed chunks of language. The best approach is to look at all of the words that occur in phrases to see if they also occur alone. A SALT-generated list of the word occurring in the sample is a useful organizing tool for this analysis. Frequent words can then be explored to see if they always occur in the same phrases. This would indicate that the child is using a more Gestalt approach.

2. **Try with school-age children.** Make a list of the three most challenging children on your caseload and the three that are the easiest to treat. How do these two groups differ from each other? How are they the same? Do your intervention plans reflect these similarities and differences? Identify an activity or approach that works well with one child and try it with another child whom you have identified as being either the same or different than the first child.

35 Cultural Differences in Parent-Child Interaction

My first real faculty position was at Indiana University in Bloomington. I had spent my entire life in California but, jobs being scarce, I suddenly found myself in Middle America. My friends at IU were frequently bemused, or amused, by my Berkeley ways and would say things like, "That's because you're from California." To which I always replied, "No, it's just me." Finally I had an epiphany: I was indeed being myself, but that self had been importantly shaped by West Coast culture. I was who I was because of the values and way of life I had grown up with, and my cultural roots were affecting my everyday activity.

The reality and importance of culture is pretty basic, but we haven't yet learned to think about it very well as interventionists. We often give parents advice about how they should interact with their children without regard for home culture. Researchers have studied contemporary Western European/North American patterns of parent-child interaction and have described them in detail. We often use this information as the basis for our advice to parents, forgetting that ours is just one of many social contexts in which children learn to talk. Ann van Kleeck (1994) reviews the cross-cultural literature and identifies four parameters of cultural difference that influence adult-child interaction: the status of children; the value of talk; the connections between social position and language dominance; and the importance of parental teaching.

Patterns of parent-child interaction differ dramatically from one ethnic group to the next, yet children around the world all learn to talk at about the same age with equal ease. The Western way seems natural to us, but it may be strange to some of the families we serve, and it certainly is not the requisite path to language.

For four years now I have been exploring cultural differences in beliefs and practices regarding adult talk to children. It seemed to me that if we knew more about alternative modes of parent-child interaction, we could adapt our practice and offer advice to families that was in better harmony with their cultures. I have come to realize that it is actually difficult, if not impossible, to view the world from a different perspective. I remain convinced, however, that if we know about cultural differences, we can do a better job of helping families find the best ways to support their child's development.

Chinese versus Western Patterns of Talk to Children

Our first project explored the ways in which Chinese and Western mothers differ in their beliefs and practices concerning interactions with young children. We (Johnston & Wong, 2002) prepared a questionnaire in English or Chinese that was distributed to mothers by staff members at local health agencies. The survey asked respondents to indicate their level of agreement with 20 belief statements (e.g., Young children learn important things while playing) and also to indicate the frequency with which they used 12 verbal interaction practices (e.g., Ask my child to repeat a sentence after me).

Responses from 42 Chinese mothers and 44 Western mothers were ultimately analyzed. Statistical tests indicated that, taken together, ratings on six belief statements or on five interaction patterns could identify members of the two groups with a high degree of accuracy. Table 35.1 indicates the percentage of mothers in each group who *agreed* or *strongly agreed* with a belief statement, and Table 35.2 indicates the percentage of mothers who reported using an interaction strategy *very often* or *almost always*.

Table 35.1   **Beliefs Identified which Cultural Membership**

Statement of Belief	% Chinese Mothers Agreed	% Western Mothers Agreed
Children learn best with instruction.	91	39
Children should be encouraged to use words…rather than gestures.	93	61
Older family members give good advice about child development.	71	36
Parental use of baby talk impedes language growth.	26	43
Young children learn important things while playing.	86	100
Young children should be allowed to join in adult conversations with nonfamily members.	50	86

Table 35.2

**Discourse Practices which
Identified Cultural Membership**

Discourse Practice	% Chinese Mothers Used	% Western Mothers Used
Read a book to their child at bedtime	29	84
Talk with their child about nonshared events	52	91
Expand their child's utterances	43	75
Prompt personal event narratives	21	73
Use picture books and flash cards to teach new words	64	46

Chinese Mothers' Beliefs and Discourse Practices

These results point to important cultural differences of two sorts. First, the Chinese mothers were much less likely to report that they often prompt their young child for personal narratives, talk with the child about nonshared events of the day, or allow the child to converse with adults who are not family members. Such activities would treat the child as a potentially equal conversational partner and, hence, reflect an expectation for independence and early verbal competence. These are not the child-rearing goals of Chinese parents, who instead value social interdependence and typically hold modest performance expectations for preschoolers (Chao, 1995).

The second area of cultural difference concerns instruction and learning. Response patterns on the belief items are consonant with the Chinese emphasis on "nurture" rather than "nature." Parents expect not only to teach children what is morally and socially right, but also to be active participants in all aspects of learning. We'll return to the Chinese data a bit later, but first some views of a second non-Western culture.

Indo-Canadian versus Western Mothers

In our most recent project we have been learning from families who emigrated from India, primarily the Punjab region. Our primary data again came from written surveys, this time completed by 52 Indo-Canadian mothers and 47 Euro-Canadian mothers of preschool-age children. We distributed the surveys in

English, Hindi, or Punjabi through community health centers and cultural organizations. The questionnaire was structured much like the one in the earlier project but the questions were specific to the Indian cultures.

Analysis of the survey responses indicated that there were significant group differences on 14 of the belief items and 9 of the verbal interaction practice items. If we considered the items as a set, we could again predict the culture of each mother with high accuracy (Simmons & Johnston, 2003).

Indian Mothers' Beliefs

Table 35.3 lists some of the belief items showing large differences between cultures. I've grouped them thematically and indicated the percentage of mothers who *agreed* or *strongly agreed* with the statement.

Table 35.3 **Beliefs More Typical of Indian Mothers**

Statement of Belief	Indian Culture	European Culture
Children usually ask too many questions.	83	13
Mothers should always fulfill their children's wishes and try to keep them happy.	41	17
The most important thing for young children is to learn about family relationships and expectations.	70	33
Children who can follow directions probably know how to talk.	62	18
When children make errors in their speech, parents should correct them.	89	63

Each survey item taps into a complicated set of beliefs and values. And, in the case of India, our understanding is further challenged by great cultural variation *within* the country. To help us interpret the data, we invited a group of seven professional women from within our local Indian community to meet with us and comment on the survey responses. The ensuing discussion assisted us in discerning three themes in the data.

Answers to the first two items reflect the **importance of children.** At first this value seems incompatible with the view that *children ask too many questions*. The strong agreement with this item initially suggested to me a certain disregard for young children or perhaps a sense that children should be seen and not heard. As it turned out, I had totally misjudged the social context and interaction patterns that give rise to this opinion. My cultural informants explained that Indian mothers always stop what they are doing and attend to their children when they ask for attention, assistance, or information. This is true even if the mothers are busy with work or talking with someone else. As one woman explained, "There is no such thing as 'my time' or an 'adult conversation.' The needs of the children come first." Given this priority one might indeed feel that children have too many questions!

Responses to the next item indicate the **importance of family,** but if my panelists are at all typical, a better index of this value might be the phone bill. I heard many stories of birthday calls to India and other efforts to maintain the bonds within extended families. Family members are referred to by relationship (e.g., father's brother) rather than first names, and are seen as more important than friends. One panelist talked about both the pressures and the security that result from the importance of family. Family members receive respect and support, but everything that one does is seen to reflect back on family.

Responses to the last two items in Table 35.2 reflect an interesting combination of the first two that I will call **being parents.** Indian mothers tend to believe that *if a child can follow directions he probably knows how to talk*. The large group differences on this item do not necessarily indicate some greater knowledge of language acquisition among Western parents. Instead, my panelists looked beyond the particular domain to general beliefs about children's learning. They saw Indian parents as being more optimistic about their children than Western parents, more confident that all would be well. The quiet child is not seen as inadequate, merely shy and needing a bit more time to learn. On the other hand, although they do not push for high achievement in young children, Indian mothers do not leave learning to chance. They feel that it is part of their role as parents to provide models and corrections when behavior of any sort, speech included, falls short of the mark.

Indian Mothers' Verbal Interaction

How do these beliefs about being parents and children translate into verbal interaction patterns? As is true for the Chinese families as well, the really important answers to that question are unknown. Until we observe the speech addressed to Indian and Chinese children as carefully as we have observed the speech addressed to Western children, we won't fully know the discourse context in which Indian children learn to speak. What our survey data do show, however, is that there are real cultural differences in patterns of parent-child verbal interaction. Table 35.4 lists the discourse practices which were less characteristic of Indian mothers than of mothers with European heritage. The percentage values indicate mothers who reported using a practice almost always.

Table 35.4   **Discourse Practices Less Typical of Indian Mothers**

Discourse Practice	Indian Mothers	Western Mothers
Follow their preschool child's conversational topic	28	84
Read a book to their preschool child at bedtime	28	75
Ask child to relate a personal event narrative to a third party	23	51

These data indicate that Indian mothers, like the Chinese mothers, do not seek to create opportunities for conversational apprenticeship in the same way that Western families do. Children are not as often expected to take the lead in conversation nor to relate their experiences. Interestingly, the panelists again jumped to more general issues. One of them saw these Western discourse strategies as part of a larger set of attempts to promote independence and asked, "Why should a child be independent? Let children be children. If three-year-olds wish help in dressing or eating, why not give it to them?" Being healthy and happy is more important than being independent or accomplished.

The Indian mothers also resembled the Chinese mothers in not often reading to their children at bedtime, although the trend here was less dramatic. I suggested to the panel that the data could be misleading if mothers merely read at another time during the day. My cultural informants seemed quite ready, however, to accept these responses as valid, and offered two interpretations. First, there were very few children's books available in Punjabi, Hindi, or other Indian languages. Second, they said that there was a rich oral tradition in India, with parents passing on to their children the songs, poems, and stories they themselves grew up with. The bedtime story for them was an oral tale of princes and gods, told in the same way time after time.

Implications for Culturally Adapted Practice

Answers to many of the survey questions were clearly different for mothers in the Western and non-Western cultures, and these differences invite us to rethink our advice to families.

First, we have no reason to believe that Western-style interactions are the only, or best, way to support language learning. The fact that all children learn to speak at much the same age and in much the same fashion would argue otherwise. Instead of advising Chinese or Indian families to adopt Western-style interaction, we can suggest activities that would seem to have the same potential function but also to be more in line with cultural expectations. For example, for both cultures, the routines of book reading could be replaced by oral storytelling, or review of family photo albums. For Chinese families, play sessions on the floor could be replaced by more structured speech and language lessons.

Second, some of our usual advice to families may reflect Western goals of child rearing rather than the needs of language learning. Indian and Chinese families may not wish, or expect, young children to be independent and equal conversational partners, preferring instead to emphasize social interdependence. We may need to forget about dinner table reports of the day's events, and respect a different version of childhood. We will also need to be culture-smart when we see four-year-olds who need help with dressing or toileting. A given behavior may indicate social-emotional immaturity in one culture and be perfectly ordinary in another.

Exploring Culture

Cultural diversity is not something to be ignored or regretted. If it makes our professional lives a bit more complex, it also invites us to listen to and to appreciate the many ways of being human—including our own. You may not have a large Indian or Chinese community near your workplace or home, but I would bet that there is some local cultural community that you would like to understand. Perhaps my experience with Chinese and Indian families can be of some use. If you would like to do your own cultural explorations using surveys or interviews, here are some steps I have found useful:

1. Find someone in the cultural community who will be your research partner.

2. Start with library research to get a general idea of key beliefs and values.

3. Talk to other professionals who work with families in the community (e.g., SLPs, social workers, teachers). Invite a group for coffee and ask them for stories.

4. Create a pool of possible questions and invite members of the community to meet with you and discuss whether the questions are clear and relevant. More tea and coffee.

5. If you translate the survey into another language, be sure to add the back-translation step. Have a second translator turn the text back into English to provide an important opportunity to check the equivalency of the two texts.

6. Distribute your surveys or schedule in-depth interviews with client families.

7. Organize your findings.

8. Invite members of the cultural community to meet and help you interpret the findings. This will be particularly important with survey data. Keep in mind the comment of one of my students who wisely observed, "Maybe they do it for some other reason." More coffee.

9. Invite a group of SLPs to talk over the clinical implications of what you have learned. Wine this time?

10. Share your new practice ideas with other professionals in newsletters, workplace discussion groups, posters, and conference presentations.

The Larger Lessons

As well as learning about specific cultural differences and methods of inquiry, my colleagues and I are learning to think about cultural competence in a more nuanced fashion. Perhaps some of these broader reflections will be useful to you as you think further about our findings and your own investigations.

- **Avoid stereotypes.** Our results merely indicate questions to raise and issues to explore as we collaborate with Chinese families. No one family is completely and perfectly Chinese or Indian—or Western.

- **Look beyond behavior.** It is ultimately the culture-based meaning of a behavior that is important. The same parental behavior can have very different meanings in different cultural contexts. Feeding a three-year-old could indicate impatience or acceptance. Directiveness could imply coercion and control, or loving concern.

- **Remember our ignorance.** Our survey studies began with a picture of Western child-directed talk and showed that Chinese and Indian families don't use many of these patterns. Unfortunately, we could not explore the unique ways that parents in these non-Western cultures do interact with young children because these are as yet unknown. As future research reveals these patterns, we can further refine our intervention practice.❖

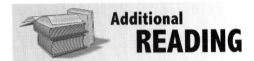

Additional
READING

Chao, R. (1995). Beyond parental control and authoritarian parenting style: Understanding Chinese parenting through the cultural notion of training. *Child Development, 65,* 111–119.

Chaudhary, N. (1999). Language socialization: Patterns of caregiver speech to young children. In T. S. Saraswathi (Ed.), *Culture, socialization, and human development: Theory, research, and applications in India* (pp. 145–166). Thousand Oaks, CA: Sage.

Early Childhood Research Institute (www.clas.uiuc.edu) *Culturally and Linguistically Appropriate Service.*

van Kleeck, A. (1994). Potential cultural bias in training parents as conversational partners with their children who have delays in language development. *American Journal of Speech-Language Pathology, 3*(1), 67–78.

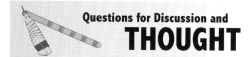

Questions for Discussion and
THOUGHT

1. What is the largest non-Western culture group in your region? What do you know about the culture of this group? van Kleeck (1994) discusses the sorts of cultural difference that will affect the social contexts in which children learn to talk. These include differences in the status of children, the value of talk, the connections between social position and language dominance, and the importance of parental teaching. Can you describe the beliefs and practices of your local non-Western communities in each of these areas?

2. What changes do you make in your practice when you have a client family or school child from these groups?

3. Does the whole idea of culturally adapted practice make sense to you? What values, learning theories, and educational goals are implicit in this idea?

4. How would you describe your own beliefs and practices regarding talk to children?

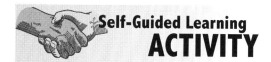

Self-Guided Learning
ACTIVITY

Choose a culture group from among those in your area. Arrange for a consultation session with a member of that community. This could be a parent, a teacher's aide, a daycare worker, or a staff member in the community center. Talk with this person about the values and practices that are typical of families in the culture. It is very likely that this person will already have thought about cultural differences and will appreciate the opportunity to share his or her views.

36 Bilingual Expectations

My father's first language was Swedish and I remember as a child thinking it was sad that he no longer spoke it. That was about as close to bilingualism as I got— that and the sound of my grandmother's accent which is tied in memory to a welcoming smile and great cookies. I don't think I would ever have been a fluent bilingual speaker, but these days in particular I regret my limited language experience. My world is full of people who speak in both of the official languages of Canada, or in Punjabi, Hindi, Tagalog, Farsi, Mandarin, Shuswap, Arabic, Cantonese—the list can get very long. Data from the U.S. Census 2000 (U.S. Census Bureau; www.factfinder.census.gov) indicate that 18.5 percent of children ages 5 to 17 do not speak English at home, but also that 87 percent of these children speak English "well" or "very well." Bilingualism is becoming a reality in the United States. Here in Canada, diversity reigns. The 2001 Census data (www40.statcan.ca) indicate that 37 percent of Vancouver residents and 18 percent of all Canadians have neither French nor English as their mother tongue. In fact, 4.7 percent of Vancouver residents have no knowledge of either of these languages. At one local rehab center, client families speak more than 23 different languages! As a result of trends such as these, SLPs and other educators are increasingly asked to decide whether a child with limited proficiency in a second language is disordered or merely bilingual. How do we decide? This is a special challenge for people like me, who have little experience on which to base our expectations.

Fortunately there are a few researchers in our field who are true polyglots and do know what to expect. One of these persons is Elin Thordardottir, an Icelandic woman who grew up in Paris and earned her higher degrees in English. Now at McGill University in Montreal, Thordardottir is encouraging us to rethink the profession's traditional views on bilingualism by looking at different sorts of bilingual therapy, observing bilingual learners, and developing new assessment tools.

One Language or Two?

For decades, language therapists have been advising families that children with learning disorders should only learn one language, usually the language of schooling and/or power. We have done so with little awareness of the difficulty or implications of following this advice: parents unable to speak with their children, children isolated from family affairs, constraints on a family's natural patterns of code-switching, disrupted relationships with members of the extended family, lost opportunities for communication (and hence, ironically, for language learning). The amazing thing in retrospect is that we also gave this advice in the virtual absence of supportive research.

Fortunately, not all families have listened. Thordardottir (2002) interviewed the parents of 10 children with Down syndrome about their views on this issue. She found that although 8 of the 10 families had been advised by professionals to limit their child's language learning to one language, only 3 had actually done so. Many had conducted their own research on the topic and had heard of or met children with learning impairments who were successfully bilingual. This evidence, coupled with their belief that bilingualism would be crucial for life success, led them to disregard the professional advice.

Tackling this issue in a different way, Thordardottir et al. (1997) report a case study that compares two approaches to language therapy with a young bilingual child. The child, S.P., came to the United States from Iceland at 30 months of age. At that time, his parents noted delays in his acquisition of Icelandic and he was seen for three months of therapy in that language. His therapy then switched to English since an Icelandic-speaking SLP was no longer available. He was also enrolled in an English-language daycare program. The family anticipated being in the United States through the first few years of S.P.'s schooling and wanted him to learn English, but since they intended to return to Iceland it was also important that his first language be maintained.

Thordardottir's observations of S.P. began at 59 months of age. At that point his English MLU was 2.52, and his PPVT score was at the 1st percentile. Icelandic was his preferred language at home, but his knowledge of that language was also significantly delayed. The therapy experiment focused on vocabulary learning, and contrasted two different approaches. Two sets of eight words were selected as learning targets, one for each approach. Twice-weekly sessions were conducted using one or the other approach in random order. In approach #1, the new words were presented only in English, and S.P.'s Icelandic utterances were not answered in Icelandic. Instead, he was reminded that a second adult in the room did not understand Icelandic and he would need to speak English. In approach #2, all of S.P.'s utterances were expanded in whichever language he chose to speak and the new words were presented in both languages. The second adult in the room for these sessions did speak Icelandic.

By the end of seven weeks, probe tasks indicated that S.P. was producing most of the 16 words. There was no difference in the number of words learned in the two approaches overall. However, for words likely to be used at home (e.g., *mittens, socks, powder, brush)* rather than at school (e.g., *string, crayon, triangle, felt)*, the bilingual approach led to somewhat earlier learning. The most important finding here is really the absence of difference. That is, for a family that was committed to bilingualism, it was important to learn that their decision was not impeding their child's vocabulary learning.

As an aside, it is worth noting here that one of the most heated debates about bilingual education, especially in the United States, concerns the degree to which the child's first language should be used in instruction. At one end of the continuum, immersion programs teach only in L2; at the other end of the continuum, bilingual programs explicitly balance the languages of instruction, trying to use L1 to facilitate the learning of, and in, L2. The two approaches to language therapy in the Thordardottir et al. (1997) case study exactly mirror this contrast. See The Language Policy Website & Emporium (http://ourworld.compuserve.com/homepages/JWCRAWFORD) for much thought-provoking material on this and related issues.

Bilingual Preschoolers

In a third recent study, Thordardottir et al. (2003) compared the English-language competencies of 11 monolingual preschoolers and 7 French-English bilingual preschoolers who had essentially equal exposure to both languages in interactive contexts. All of the children were developing normally according to their parents, and all earned nonverbal IQ scores within the normal range. The groups also did not differ in age (2;6 to 3) or in level of maternal education (17 years). The researchers used the PPVT and the Reynell to assess language skills normatively, calculated MLU from a language sample, and asked parents to complete the CDI. On all of the English language measures except the PPVT, the bilingual preschoolers earned significantly and substantially lower scores, and even the PPVT gap was large. Mean raw scores on the Reynell were 41.6 versus 31, on the PPVT were 41 versus 24, and mean MLUs were 3.36 versus 2.52.

These findings do not mean that the bilingual preschoolers had been less successful as language learners overall, since they had also been learning French. In fact, several recent studies have documented the distributed nature of an early bilingual lexicon (e.g., Lin & Johnson, 2005) with many words known in only one or the other of the child's languages. But these data can inform our expectations. The families in this project lived and worked in a highly bilingual city and were obviously well educated. They could be expected to value bilingualism in their children, to present positive models of bilingual competence, and to provide supportive language learning environments. Nevertheless, at age 3 these preschoolers were far behind the monolingual children in their knowledge of English. We can expect this gap to close as the children approach school age. Better longitudinal research, with larger samples and more demographic diversity, is needed to tell the entire story. It is clear from these and other similar data, however, that when bilingual children come to us as young preschoolers, considerable delays in English proficiency are to be expected.

In sum, our professional expectations surrounding bilingualism need updating. We must now expect more families to be bilingual and to want their children to be bilingual, even those who have learning difficulties. We must expect the challenges of somehow bringing L1 into our therapy sessions. And we must expect the pace of early language learning to look different in bilingual contexts.

A recent survey of school speech-language pathologists in Michigan (Caesar, 2005) suggests that practices have not kept pace with social change. In a sample of some 450 respondents, 75 percent said they assessed only in English, only 33 percent used informal assessment procedures, use of interpreters fell between "rarely" and "sometimes," and no one at all reported using dynamic assessment. The professional challenges of bilingualism are undeniable, but there still seems to be much room for improvement in our practice.

Local Norms

I have never been a great fan of local norms, but this year I found myself attempting to create my first local normative database. It all began with Turkish.

In the fall of 2002, a Turkish researcher named Funda Acarlar came to UBC as a visiting scholar. Dr. Acarlar taught in the special education program of Ankara University and was particularly interested in children with language problems. She and I had long conversations about the difficulties of early intervention in the absence of any standardized assessment instruments. The solution turned out to be the linguistic analysis program SALT (Miller & Iglesias, 2003–2005). The really important fact about the latest version of SALT is that you can add your own database to the program! Dr. Acarlar and I spent 2 months adapting SALT analyses to the Turkish language, and she spent the next 18 months refining the program and developing a database of some 140 language samples from children ages 3 to 6. Due to her efforts, educators and researchers in Turkey and Europe will now have a fine new tool for assessing language abilities in children learning Turkish.

With the Turkish project well underway, it occurred to me that SALT could also be an important tool in our evaluation of bilingual children here in North America. If we could create a database that represented the English competencies of the typical bilingual child, we could use it to make more informed clinical judgments. I use the word *typical* advisedly, knowing that no such child exists. Family patterns of language use, the grammar of L1, language politics and policies, differences in educational opportunities—there are many differences among bilingual communities that can influence a child's learning of a second language. Nevertheless, I thought that we could specify a database sufficiently enough to be useful, if not quite definitive, especially given the absence of alternative measures.

"How Far Have They Come?" was a collaborative project between my Child Language Lab and local school districts. Our goal was to collect language samples from bilingual children who had entered kindergarten with very limited knowledge of English and were now in October of grade 2. Additionally, the children were to be judged by their teachers as doing well in school, and by their parents as speaking their first language in an age-appropriate fashion. The intent was to create a normative database that could be used by school personnel to evaluate the progress in English of children who had been instructed in English for two years. This single snapshot of bilingual competence would be just a beginning, but hopefully a useful one for SLPs practicing in the schools.

As is always the case, the project hit a few unexpected snags. It proved difficult to find out what the relative English proficiency of bilingual children in grade 2 had been when they were kindergartners. Many children had changed schools, teachers had retired, or records had not been kept in ways that answered our questions. We nevertheless obtained 30 samples and are now compiling the database.

Local norms derived from SALT databases will never be sufficient to answer our questions about a bilingual child. But they can provide important evidence which, when coupled with other data (e.g., family or teacher concerns, developmental history, observations, information about risk factors, description of family patterns of language use, diagnostic teaching), should improve our assessment decisions. Used wisely, SALT databases will help us refine our expectations for language learning in bilingual children, or for that matter, in any group of children who are out of the mainstream.❖

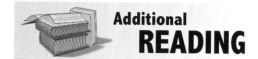

Additional
READING

Kay-Raining Bird, E., Cleave, P., Trudeau, N., Thordardottir, E., Sutton, A., & Thorpe, A. (2005). The language abilities of bilingual children with Down Syndrome. *American Journal of Speech-Language Pathology, 14,* 187–199.

Kritikos, E. (2003). Speech-language pathologists' beliefs about language assessment of bilingual/bicultural individuals. *American Journal of Speech-Language Pathology, 12,* 73–91.

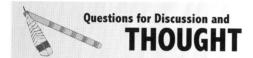

Questions for Discussion and
THOUGHT

1. Where, if at all, did you learn that children with developmental disorders should only learn one language? What was the rationale given?

2. What variables could influence a child's success in learning English as L2? Would you expect the same outcomes from an L2 immersion program if L2 was not the majority language?

3. What are your current strategies for assessing children who do not speak English as L1?

4. Imagine you were given $5,000 for a local bilingual assessment project. Which approach would you take (local norms, dynamic assessment, interpreter training and use, other)? Why? Which language(s) would you focus on? Why? How would you organize the study? Who could you get to help? Now that you have planned the study, pick up the phone and call your local service club (e.g., Rotary, Junior League, Elks, Masons). Make an appointment to talk to them about being sponsors of the study and get started.

Thinking About Child Language

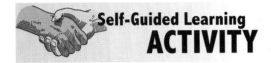

Self-Guided Learning
ACTIVITY

Put yourself in the shoes of a child learning L2. Invite someone you know who speaks another language, preferably non-Western, to serve as your language model and informant. Invite a few professional friends over for a two-hour session in which you all attempt to learn this new language. The rule is that your inform-ant cannot speak or respond to English. All exchanges with him or her must be in the new language. Bring props like old clothes and household goods. Divide into teams and plan some sort of interaction. For example, hold up objects and look quizzical, make objects do their typical things while the informant describes your actions, or invent small role-playing vignettes. At the end of an hour or so, tell your informant that he or she can now speak English, and discuss whatever hypotheses you have developed about how the language is organized. Were you on the right track? Did your first language influence your interpretations? Also, explore any communication breakdowns that may have occurred, trying to figure out what went wrong. Loosen up and have fun. I guarantee you will learn some-thing useful about language learning and bilingualism.

Before you begin, include the group in this discussion of ground rules. Ask your informant to (1) ignore pronunciation as much as possible, (2) speak to you in a simple fashion, as to a young child, and (3) be as helpful as possible—but no English.

37 Bilingualism: A Tale of Two Countries

Possibilities, Retrenchment, and Alternatives

It was the early 1970s and I was in grad school in Berkeley when I first heard the important news from Canada. Researchers at the Ontario Institute for Studies in Education had demonstrated that the school difficulties we commonly associated with instruction in a second language were not inherent in knowing and using two languages. When children were immersed in a second language that was valued by their families and were not penalized for using their first language in the classroom, they made good academic progress. This new information supported a wide range of experiments in bilingual education for the decade that followed.

Those times have come to an end in much of the United States. Incipient xenophobia, economic ills, demographic changes, and other social forces have lessened the public's commitment to bilingual education and the value placed on cultural and linguistic diversity. While it is true that the number of persons in the United States over age 5 who speak a language other than English at home has increased by half during the last decade, according to 2000 census data, this group still constitutes only 18 percent of the population and 87 percent of them also speak English "well" or "very well" (U.S. Census Bureau: http://www.factfinder.census.gov). Nevertheless, by May of 1987, half the persons queried in a *New York Times*/CBS poll agreed that there should be an "amendment to the Constitution that requires federal, state, and local governments to conduct business in English and not use other languages, even in places where many people don't speak English" (Crawford, 1997).

In 1998, California passed a law that restricted bilingual education to one year for children with limited English proficiency (LEP). Advocates of the law argued that it was the bilingual classroom that was preventing children from learning English, and predicted that the new restrictions would improve the overall English competence of school children (Crawford, 2002). Five years later, only 1 in 13 children have actually succeeded in moving out of the LEP category during their one year of intensive English instruction. Data from San Francisco (12,000 students, 1994–1995 and 1996–1997) indicate that in actuality, a child requires about four years of special language support services in order to move from LEP to Fluent English Speaker, the level of competence that best serves classroom learning (Ramirez, 1998).

Canadians, on the other hand, have long acknowledged the value of bilingualism. The percentage of Canadians whose mother tongue is neither English nor French is about 17 percent, very close to the percentage of persons in the United States whose mother tongue is not English (www40.Statcan.ca). Yet, attitudes are very different. More than 85 percent of Canadians think it is important for their child to speak a second language and are in favor of multiculturalism. And in a recent poll, some 90 percent of Canadians living outside Quebec agreed that the French Canadians in their province should have a right to education in French (Parkin & Turcotte, 2004). Here in Vancouver, only 43 percent of school children are from English-speaking homes. The province of British Columbia funds up to five years of special programming for children learning English as a second language and a full 25 percent of school enrollees take advantage of these programs (Krowchuk, 2005). These policies make good sense to me on the grounds of social justice, cross-cultural understanding, and the economic benefits of school success. Recently I learned of a further set of supporting arguments: researchers are discovering that bilingual children actually perform better than monolingual children on a variety of cognitive tasks.

The Advantages of Bilingualism

Ellen Bialystok and her colleagues at York University in Toronto have been major contributors to this line of study. Bialystok's view is that the bilingual speaker must constantly inhibit one language and that "early and massive exercise of that function appears to have generalized effects for young children," leading to a superiority in the inhibitory processes (Bialystok & Martin, 2004, p. 338). She also notes that bilingual experiences may, in some situations, result in greater cognitive flexibility.

In one recent series of experiments, monolingual English-speaking five-year-olds were compared with bilingual English-Cantonese speakers of the same age. The bilingual group all spoke Cantonese at home and earned English-language vocabulary scores at the 30th percentile or above, indicative of some considerable degree of bilingual competence. The children were given a computerized version of the Dimensional Change Card Sort. The task required the child to sort a set of pictured objects into two bins, first by one criterion, then by a different criterion.

In one condition, for example, the same set of shapes was sorted first by color, then by shape (or vice versa). In a second condition, rabbits and flowers were sorted by kind or by color. The challenging part of the task was that the cue pictures for the two bins didn't change, only the instructions changed. So, for example, in one condition a blue bunny marked the bin for blue things, then immediately following, it marked the bin for bunnies. The major finding was that bilingual children sorted more items correctly in this task.

Bialystok and Martin argue that in order to succeed in the Card Sort task, the child needed to inhibit or ignore a property than had been relevant and hold in mind an alternative interpretation. However, the researchers subsequently emphasize the demands for inhibition and gloss over what seem to me to be the equally important demands for remembering the current rule. They do, however, note that there were no group differences on a simple digit-span task, which puts the memory explanation in some doubt. Whatever the reasons, the finding of a bilingual advantage on this task is clear.

I find a second study by this group even more convincing. Bialystok et al. (in press) used the Simon Task to again look at the control of attention, both inhibition and selectivity. In this task, a square appeared on the computer screen directly above one of two response buttons. The child is told to press the red button when the square is red and the blue button when the square is blue. On *congruent* trials the color of the square matches the color of the button directly below it; on *incongruent* trials the color of the square does not match the nearest button and the child must ignore the spatial cue in favor of the color cue. The interpretation of this task seems more straightforward than the Card Sort task, since there is no need to reinterpret any cues and the response rule stays constant.

Reaction time data from five-year-old French-English bilingual children was compared with data from English monolingual children. The bilingual children had the faster times in both conditions. The researchers argue that, since the trials were randomized, even the congruent trials placed high demands on executive functions. Bialystok et al. (in press) attribute the observed differences to "some type of executive control, including both the working memory to keep focused on the rule and the inhibition to avoid executing the automatic response" (p. tba).

Thesis research by Caroline Marcoux (2004) at UBC has just replicated this finding and added weight to the interpretation. Marcoux tested some 60 children in grade 3, half of them monolingual French speakers and half of them bilingual

French-English speakers. The bilingual group had faster reaction times in the Simon Task and also performed better on an auditory working memory task requiring the reorganization and recall of noun labels.

These three studies are just a few from the growing set that point to the cognitive advantages of childhood bilingualism. Although the experimental tasks are quite artificial, there is reason to believe that these small differences in processing skill may translate into real differences in everyday problem-solving abilities. The evidence in this case again comes from San Francisco. The review of student performance data from 12,000 students in the 1994–1995 and 1996–1997 school years (Ramirez, 1998) indicates that once students who were initially classified as Limited English Proficiency become fluent English speakers, they are the highest achieving students in the district! Bilingualism does seem to be good for more than travel comforts, lectures, and civil service jobs…sometimes.

An Exception?

Not all of the research studies on cognitive processes and bilingualism report advantages. Gutierrez-Clellen et al. (2004) wanted to identify measures of verbal working memory that could differentiate children with language problems from dialect speakers and children whose first language was not the language of the test. Two tasks that had been developed for studying language processes in children with learning problems seemed like good bets: the competing language processing task (CLPT; Gaulin & Campbell, 1994) and the dual processing comprehension task (DPCT; Ellis Weismer, 1996). In the CLPT, sets of sentences are presented one at a time. The listener indicates whether or not each sentence is true. Then at the end of the set, the listener must also recall the last word of each sentence. The number of sentences in the set increases as the test proceeds. In the DPCT, the listener hears two simultaneous instructions for manipulating objects, one male voice and one female voice, and must follow both. Performance in this simultaneous condition is compared with performance on the two sets of instructions presented separately. Neither the CLPT nor the DPCT requires complex syntactic knowledge or vocabulary depth, and quasi-normative data from monolingual English speaking children are available for each.

Twenty-two Spanish-English bilingual children in grade 2 participated in the study. They were able to tell stories in each language that contained few grammatical errors, and were rated by parents and teachers at either 3 or 4 on a 4 point scale for frequency of use and proficiency in each language. The working memory capacity of these bilingual children was compared to that of an age-matched group who were proficient in only one of the languages, either Spanish or English. The findings in this study differed from those reported by Bialystok and Marcoux: the bilingual children showed no reliable superiority on either the CLPT or the DPCT.

Implications for Practice

So what happened to the bilingual cognitive advantage? There are several possibilities. First, the CLPT and the DPCT require sentence comprehension, while tasks in the other studies required only the knowledge of highly familiar nouns. So perhaps the cognitive advantage can be overridden by verbal demands. Second, the monolingual and bilingual groups may have been less distinct in the Gutierrez-Clellen et al. (2004) study than in the Canadian studies. Although not proficient in both languages, many of the children in their monolingual group had considerable experience with Spanish *and* English. Perhaps the advantage is only clear when contrasting the extreme poles of the bilingual continuum. Finally, it is worth noting that the study took place in southern California during a time when there was much negative opinion being expressed about bilingual education and the Hispanic community in particular. There may not have been the encouragement or opportunity for children to develop the strong, coordinate bilingualism that results in a cognitive advantage. If so, it seems that once again there may be social factors determining the outcomes of learning in a bilingual society.

In many communities, SLPs serve as general language development experts, and have the opportunity to advise teachers and policymakers on topics that go well beyond disorders. This is certainly not my area of strength, but thanks to my students I have been thinking and reading about bilingualism quite a bit over the last year, and have a few opinions to share should anyone ask. Here's my current bottom line:

- Bilingualism can have positive cognitive consequences, but these are most likely to occur in children with strong, coordinate bilingualism, that is, where both languages are learned at the same time, from an early age, and used daily.

- It takes more time to learn a second language during the school years than we initially thought, at least if the goal is the high level of proficiency needed for successful classroom learning.

- The relative performance of bilingual children on verbal working memory tasks can be quite varied, depending on the nature of the language required.

More data are needed before these measures can provide a reliable alternative to traditional language tests.

- The social climate is a key determinant of the outcomes of bilingual education because it can affect program availability and the acceptability of knowing and using nonmajority languages.❖

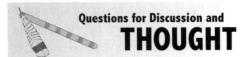

Questions for Discussion and
THOUGHT

1. What criteria could you use to decide whether a child's competencies in two languages were equivalent? Especially if there are no standardized tests in one of the languages?

2. How do the general conclusions in this essay translate into advice to parents? Teachers? Educational policymakers in your locale? What is the current state of local programming for students with LEP? Are there opportunities for advocacy?

3. Draw up a parent interview protocol you could use to explore language usage patterns at home? Which questions might parents be reluctant to answer? Keep in mind that open-ended questions are likely to garner the best information, and avoid the approach of phone survey takers who are anxious to have you choose one of their expected answers.

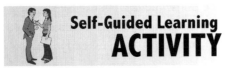

Self-Guided Learning
ACTIVITY

Invite a parent of a bilingual child on your caseload to join you for coffee (or whatever is appropriate and socially inviting) and talk about the language usage patterns in their home. Who uses what languages with whom, for what topics? What languages are in printed materials? Do they talk about language learning and loss? What are their aspirations and fears? Listen carefully and be the learner.

38 Vive la Différence

My introduction to developmental psychology came in a Stanford course taught by Eleanor Maccoby. Although her rigor and uncompromising demeanor left me more than a little anxious around exam time, her expertise was clear—even to a novice. What I didn't fully appreciate at the time was that Maccoby was also a ground-breaking scientist who was establishing the new territory of gender-role socialization.

The topic of sex-linked differences in ability or achievement has cycled in and out of favor several times since those days, as the emphasis in developmental psychology has swung between nature and nurture. We now recognize that there are innate cognitive differences between men and women, but also that the biological differences mature in a social arena with strong gender role expectations. As is always the case, these environmental influences can mitigate or enhance one's native abilities.

Language development seems to provide the textbook case of this interaction. Girls do have a slight edge in starting to talk, but the differences seen in older children are primarily the result of social forces. For years, I have downplayed the magnitude of gender differences in language development and have believed that they had little importance for assessment or intervention planning with young children. A new study from Minnesota has reawakened my interest in this topic.

Differences in Early Vocabulary Development

A group of researchers at the University of Minnesota's Institute of Child Development has just published a longitudinal study of early vocabulary growth, looking particularly at words that are gender-typed (Stennes et al., 2005). Their method was straightforward. They asked a panel of judges to rate each word listed in CDI according to whether it was "stereotypically associated with feminine gender concepts or masculine gender concepts" (p. 77). From these data, 16 words were identified as strongly feminine (e.g., *beads, necklace, girl, dress, gentle)* and another 16 as strongly masculine (e.g., *fire truck, hammer, man, cowboy)*. They then looked for these words in CDI data they had collected from the parents of 52 children (26 girls, 26 boys) over a two-year span, at 13, 18, 24, 30, and 36 months of age.

Thinking About Child Language

The results were quite startling, at least to me. By the age of 24 months, children were already showing gender-related differences in the words they produced. Boys were more likely to be using the masculine gender-typed words, and girls the feminine ones. This remained true even when the researchers statistically controlled for overall vocabulary size. But that's not all. When the researchers looked at the CDI data for even younger children they found more gender-linked differences—this time in gestures. At 13 and 18 months, it was the boys who were more likely to pretend to dig with a shovel or pound with a hammer, and the girls who were more likely to burp the baby doll or wipe its face. Again, this difference remained when the researchers controlled for total number of symbolic gestures.

By 36 months, the observed differences in gender-typed words or gestures on the CDI were fading as more and more of the children reached ceiling on this list. Their existence during the preceding years is nevertheless eye opening. I was used to thinking about peer influences on vocabulary during the later preschool years. I can still see the swarms of junior Batmen swishing their capes as they ran through our classroom. But one- and two-year-olds!

Differences in Play and Parental Language Input

As I read the Stennes et al. (2005) discussion, however, I quickly realized that there were many possible roots for these early vocabulary and gesture differences—things as simple as bedroom décor. It turns out that researchers have documented the unsurprising fact that girls' and boys' bedrooms have different appearances and contents. Girls' rooms have more dolls, more items for doll care, and more ruffles; boys' rooms have more vehicles and art materials. (My lack of surprise is just one more indication of how ingrained the gender role influences really are.)

These various objects, of course, are associated with activities, and the activities are associated with ways of talking. In a study by O'Brien and Nagle (1987), for example, parents talked quite differently with their children when they played with the toys that were gender-typed than when they played with toys that were more neutral. When playing with dolls, parents used more labeling, longer utterances, more questions, and greater lexical diversity. When playing with trucks and cars, parents used simpler sentences and spoke less often. These differences were true regardless of the genders of the parent or the child. Other researchers have found parallel differences in communicative function. Role-playing activities, more typical of girls, are likely to involve more cooperative communication and descriptive language. Construction activities (e.g., block building), more typical of boys, are likely to involve more instrumental language.

The idea that gender-role expectations can be seen in room décor and Christmas toys was scarcely news. I, after all, was once the four-year-old girl who really wanted her brother's cowboy outfit. What I hadn't stopped to think about was the language-learning implications of all those trucks and ruffles. Much of the time the differences may not be apparent. Gender takes a back seat in conversations about spilling juice or naptime. But when we think about the total corpus of language that a child hears, or about the particular salience of playtime conversations with a parent or older sibling, it is easier to see how gender expectations could influence language learning. Little girls or boys are more likely to hear, learn, and exercise certain language patterns because of the activities that they are encouraged to pursue.

Differences in Why and How Much We Talk

A recent meta-analysis (Leaper & Smith, 2004) attempts to assess the cumulative effects of gender role expectations on the development of patterns of language use. (A meta-analysis uses statistical procedures to combine the results from many studies into one grand test of significance and effect size.) Taking a page from Deborah Tannen (1990), the analyses focused on three language patterns that are strongly gender-typed: talkativeness, affiliative speech, and assertive speech.

The review covered more than 73 studies which together involved more than 5000 children, primarily between the ages of 2 and 12 years. The general finding was that, yes, girls are more talkative than boys and use more affiliative language. And, also as expected, boys use more assertive language. However—and this is a huge however—the size of the overall effects were small to negligible.

What was much more interesting was that gender differences, sometimes sizable, were more likely to be seen in certain contexts than in others. Here's a sampling:

- Girls were more talkative than boys, only in the preschool years.

- The difference in talkativeness between girls and boys was larger in conversations with adults than with peers.

- The major reason girls were more affiliative was because they were more responsive to their conversational partner, not because they were praised or acknowledged more often.

- Boys and girls become more similar in their communication patterns during the grade school years.

- Girls were especially likely to use affiliative speech when they could choose their own activities.

- The major reason that boys were more assertive was because they used more directive utterances, not because they were negative or requested information more often.

In short, the most general findings are ultimately misleading. The language that children use depends on how old they are, what they are doing, who they are talking to, and what exactly they are trying to accomplish with words.

Gender-Typed Language and Intervention

We sometimes think too narrowly about the research that supports our professional decisions. It isn't just the clinical literature on outcomes that is pertinent. As I read these two studies, I could think of many ways to use this evidence on gender differences in the practice of speech-language pathology.

As Fey (1986) pointed out many years ago, it is difficult, if not impossible, to help a child learn language if the child doesn't talk. Undue reticence can be a real therapeutic challenge. Leaper and Smith (2004) make it clear that we shouldn't conclude too quickly that boys who are not talkative are just being boys. If they are preschoolers, some degree of reticence may be expected in interactions with adults, but this would not be expected for a school-age child. In both cases, we can observe interactions with peers to confirm or disconfirm our sense that a child is not sufficiently talkative.

Secondly, it seems that we have a real opportunity during the school years to help children build good conversational skills. Leaper and Smith (2004) point out that these are the years when gender thinking is the most flexible. The initial period of gender identity has passed, and the angst of adolescence has yet to arrive. Boys can afford to be more responsive and less assertive; girls can practice topic control in ways that feel comfortable (e.g., with suggestions and information). The only programs I know about that directly tackle conversational skill do so with preadolescents and adolescents. This may be tantamount to swimming upstream.

Finally, these articles both demonstrate the influence of the activity context on the language we use. This issue has primarily appeared in the clinical literature in guidelines for obtaining the best sample of a child's language. What struck me this time was that we could also use this information to plan therapy activities and advise families. If playing house invites the use of language that is more conversationally responsive, more descriptive, and more complex, what we need are more dolls and fewer trucks.

At face value this is a ridiculous recommendation—at least for boys. Stennes et al. (2005) has convinced me that we can't ignore the realities of gender socialization. But as a metaphor, "more dolls and fewer trucks" works splendidly. We can think about the features of playing house that are language enhancing, and then create ways to incorporate these same features into the play world of little boys. It seems to me that playing house works because it utilizes familiar scripts, welcomes collaborative narrative, invites role playing, and is inherently interactive. We can create comparable activity settings with Transformer® toys, with superheroes, with Lego® cars driving children to school and home again. These toys will, I think, be perceived as gender appropriate, but—if used well—will also provide good opportunities for language learning.❖

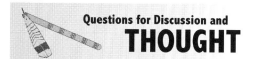

Questions for Discussion and
THOUGHT

1. If a similar study were done with adults, would we find the same sorts of connections between the activity context and the language used? Why and why not?

2. How would you respond if parents were to express their displeasure with the toys you were using with their child, saying that they were not right for a girl or boy?

3. Would you expect children with language delays to be more like their age peers or more like their language peers in regard to gender differences?

4. The essays in this section consider culture, gender, bilingualism, and learning style as variables that affect individual language learning and use. Can you think of still other dimensions of individual difference and predict their effect on language and language learning?

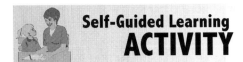

**Self-Guided Learning
ACTIVITY**

Collect two language samples from one child, using two different sets of play materials: (1) construction toys (e.g., blocks and cars for boys; art collages and blocks for girls) and (2) role playing toys (e.g., superheroes for boys; family dolls for girls). If possible, have a colleague, assistant, or family member actually interact with the child—someone who hasn't read this essay. Analyze and compare the two samples. What is different and what is the same? Look at features such as MLU, speech act functions, syntactic complexity, and turn length.

Cross-Reference Chart of Essay Contents

Section	Using Research				SLI						Auditory Perception			Assessment						
Number	1	2	3	4	5	6	7	8	9	10	11	12	13	14	15	16	17	18	19	20
Shortened Title	Language Development	Evidence	What Works	Don't Add Up	Study of SLI	Morphology Gene	Language Formulation	Memory Lessons	Being Smart	Never a Poet	Crash-Test Dummy	CAPD	Listen Up!	Fact, Fashion, Funding	Diagnostic Categories	Old Dog, New Tricks	Dynamic Assessment	To Test or Not	Another Story	Narrative Schemes
Preschool*	•																			
School-Age*					•			•	•			•	•			•				
Syntax	•				•	•										•	•			
Morphology	•				•	•	•									•				
Vocabulary	•															•				
Pragmatics																		•	•	•
Perception	•								•		•	•	•							
Intelligence					•			•	•							•				
Cognitive Processes	•					•	•	•	•			•	•			•	•	•		•
Cognitive Prerequisites	•							•												
Developmental Theory	•			•					•	•	•					•		•		
Comprehension												•		•						
Production						•	•					•							•	
Imaging, Neuroevidence						•									•					
Assessment				•								•		•	•	•	•	•	•	•
Intervention		•	•								•		•							
Families					•	•			•											
Methodology		•	•		•								•			•				
Autism				•											•					
SLI					•	•	•	•	•	•						•				

Continued on next page

Appendix A—*Cont.*

Section	Intervention Theory				Intervention Range						Vocabulary			Diversity				
Number	21	22	23	24	25	26	27	28	29	30	31	32	33	34	35	36	37	38
Shortened Title	Fit, Focus, Functionality	Reinforcement	ABA Revisited	Learn to Learn	Grammar Books	One, Two, Shoe	Best Route to Reading	Sharing Our Knowledge	Animal Charades	Blackbirds and Fiddlers	Skin of Thought	Inflections to Boot	Verb Learning	Everybody's Different	Cultural Differences	Bilingual Expectations	Bilingualism Tale	Vive la Difference
Preschool*	•			•					•	•								•
School-Age*	•			•		•			•	•	•							
All Ages*		•	•			•		•				•	•	•	•	•	•	
Syntax	•				•					•				•				
Morphology	•				•													
Vocabulary	•			•						•	•	•	•					
Pragmatics	•		•												•			
Perception									•	•				•				
Intelligence						•												
Cognitive Processes				•		•		•	•	•				•		•	•	
Cognitive Prerequisites	•		•															
Developmental Theory	•	•	•	•		•			•	•		•	•	•	•			•
Comprehension				•				•										
Production									•	•								•
Imaging, Neuroevidence																		
Assessment	•													•				
Intervention	•	•	•	•	•	•	•	•	•	•	•	•	•	•	•	•	•	•
Families						•			•	•	•					•	•	•
Methodology			•														•	
Autism		•	•						•									
SLI									•	•								

*All of the essays include material suitable for all developmental stages. If a particular age range is marked it means that the essay has sections with particular relevance to that age range.

List of Websites Cited

The following websites are cited in various essays and are listed here for convenience.

www.unl.edu/buros/

BUROS Center for Testing

Extensive archive of reviews of standardized tests. Purchase cost per review unless accessing database from university library.

www.bamford-lahey.org

Bamford-Lahey Children's Foundation

A growing bibliography of articles about language disorders and treatment; also several video presentations about Fast ForWord.

www.campbellcollaboration.org

The Campbell Collaboration

International organization concerned with the preparation of systematic reviews of educational practice.

www.cebm.net

Centre for Evidence-Based Medicine

The Oxford University center for evidence-based medicine; good tutorials.

www.cebm.utoronto.ca

Centre for Evidence-Based Medicine

Good resource for general understanding of evidence-based practice, especially the section entitled "Practicing EBM."

www.cfw.tufts.edu

Tufts University Child & Family Web Guide

An excellent gateway to reliable web-based information.

www.clas.uiuc.edu

Culturally & Linguistically Appropriate Services

A website of the Early Childhood Research Institute.

http://ourworld.compuserve.com/homepages/JWCRAWFORD

Language Policy Website & Emporium

Information on language policies and bilingual education.

Thinking About Child Language

www40.statcan.ca
Canadian Statistics
Summary tables providing an overview of Canada's people, economy, and governments.

curry.edschool.virginia.edu/go/wil/rimes_and_rhymes.htm
A Rhyme a Week: Nursery Rhymes for Early Literacy
Nursery rhyme activities for downloading.

www.languageanalysislab.com
Language Analysis Lab
Information about the SALT computer program.

www.ling.hawaii.edu/faculty/ann/
Ann Peters's Home Page
Downloadable copy of Ann Peter's book *The Units of Language Acquisition*. Contains an excellent discussion of Gestalt language learning.

www-personal.umich.edu/~pfa/dreamhouse/nursery/rhymes.html
The Mother Goose Pages
Words to many nursery rhymes.

www.psy.pdx.edu/PsiCafe/
The PSI Cafe
Resource material on many psychological theorists; see section on Piaget.

www.sci.sdsu.edu/cdi
MacArthur-Bates Communicative Development Inventory
Information about these inventories, especially norms.

www.storynet.org
Story Net
Materials for narrative activities.

www.superkids.com
SuperKids® Education for the Future
Reviews of educational software.

http://w-w-c.org
What Works Clearinghouse
Reports on the effectiveness of educational interventions. Funded and administered by the U.S. Department of Education.

http://factfinder.census.gov
U.S. Census Bureau
Factsheets and searchable database of U.S. census data.

Standardized Tests and Other Assessment Tools: Brief Descriptions and Publishers

Language

CELF	**Clinical Evaluation of Language Fundamentals** Semel, E., Wiig, E., & Secord, W. San Antonio, TX: Psychological Corp. Receptive tasks include sentence comprehension and recognizing word meaning similarities; expressive tasks include formulating sentences from given words and word association.
DSS	**Developmental Sentence Score** Lee, L. Evanston, IL: Northwestern University Press. A standardized scoring system for language samples.
EOWPVT	**Expressive One-Word Picture Vocabulary Test** Gardner, M. F. Austin, TX: Pro-Ed. Picture naming.
EVT	**Expressive Vocabulary Test** Williams, K. Austin, TX: Pro-Ed. Picture naming and provision of synonyms. Designed for comparison with PPVT.
IPSyn	**Index of Productive Syntax** Scarborough, H. S. (1990). *Applied Psycholinguistics, 11*, 1–22. A developmental coding scheme for quantifying language sample data. Norms are psychometrically weak with very few subjects in comparison group. Nevertheless useful for toddlers.
CDI	**MacArthur-Bates Communicative Development Inventories** Fenson, L., Dale, P., Reznick, J. S., Thal, D., Bates, E., Hartung, J., et al. Baltimore: Brookes. Lists from which parents select words, gestures, and phrases that child understands or says; lexical norms online; two versions: Infants-Toddlers and Early Preschool.

PPVT   **Peabody Picture Vocabulary Test**
Dunn, L., & Dunn, L.
Circle Pines, MN: American Guidance Services.
Comprehension of single word vocabulary; picture pointing;
mostly labels for concrete objects and events.

REYNELL   **Reynell Developmental Language Scales**
Reynell, J., & Gruber, C.
Los Angeles: Western Psychological Services.
Developed in Great Britain and is more commonly used there.
Yields omnibus scores for language comprehension (R) and
production (E).

SALT   **Systematic Analysis of Language Transcripts**
See Appendix D.

SICD   **Sequenced Inventory of Communication Development**
Hedrick, D., Prather, E., & Tobin, A.
Austin, TX: Pro-Ed.
Combines probe, observation, and parent report items; toddler
and early preschool; broad and diverse sampling of language
performance.

TELD   **Test of Early Language Development**
Hresko, W., Reid, K., & Hammel, D.
Austin, TX: Pro-Ed. Mixture of items. Yields three general
scores: expressive, receptive, and overall.

TLT   **The Listening Test**
Barrett, M., Huisingh, R., Bowers, L., LoGuidice, M., & Orman, J.
East Moline, IL: LinguiSystems.
Text comprehension with subscores for tasks such as extracting
the main idea, making inferences, or drawing conclusions that
go beyond the immediate information.

TNL   **Test of Narrative Language**
Gillam, R., & Pearson, N.
Austin, TX: Pro-Ed.
Three narratives to comprehend and answer questions about;
three narratives to create and tell. Series progresses from
retelling to telling with picture sequence to telling with single
picture.

TOAL	**Test of Adolescent and Adult Language**
	Hammill, D., Brown, V., Larsen, S., & Wiederholt, J. L.
	Austin, TX: Pro-Ed.
	Tests a range of language use in listening, speaking, reading, and writing tasks; grammar and vocabulary.

TOLD	**Test of Language Development**
	Newcomer, P., & Hammill, D.
	Austin, TX: Pro-Ed.
	Nine subtests with separate and composite norms; tasks include sentence comprehension, sentence repetition, provision of inflectional morphology, picture naming, and pointing to given single words.

TTFC	**Token Test for Children**
	DiSimoni, F.
	Austin, TX: Pro-Ed.
	Sentence comprehension and information processing; series of items such as "put the white circle under the blue square."

Nonverbal Cognition, Academic Achievement, & Social Skills

CMMS	**Columbia Mental Maturity Scale**
	Burgomeiser, B., Blum, L., & Lorge, I.
	San Antonio, TX: Psychological Corp.
	Nonverbal reasoning; odd item out, and visual analogy; no language use required; norms are outdated and somewhat generous; extends to older preschoolers.

LIPS	**Leiter International Performance Scale**
	Roid, G., & Miller, L.
	London: nferNelson.
	Nonverbal reasoning; 1995 'revision' very different than original. Original consisted of perceptual and conceptual matching tasks; no language use required; extends to older preschoolers.

PIAT	**Peabody Individual Achievement Test**
	Markwardt, F.
	Circle Pines, MN: American Guidance Services.
	Academic achievement in reading, spelling, math; included comprehension of written sentences, writing a story about a picture; oral reading.

Ravens   **Ravens Progressive Matrices**
Raven, J.
London: The Test Agency.
Nonverbal reasoning; select picture that completes a series; no
language use required.

TONI   **Test of Nonverbal Intelligence**
Brown, L., Sherbenou, R., & Johnsen, S.
Circle Pines, MN: American Guidance Services.
Nonverbal reasoning and problem solving; no language use
required; primary grades through adults.

Vineland   **Vineland Adaptive Behavior Scales**
Sparrow, S., Balla, D., & Cicchetti, D.
Circle Pines, MN: American Guidance Services.
Structured interview and questionnaire formats; personal and
social skills for everyday living: communication, daily living,
socialization, and motor domains.

WISC   **Wechsler Intelligence Scales for Children**
Wechsler, D.
San Antonio, TX: Psychological Corp.
One of the most widely used intelligence tests for school-age
children. Fourth edition yields scores for Perceptual Reasoning,
Verbal, Working Memory, and Processing Speed. Requires
special training to administer.

NOTE: Publication dates for tests are not listed because of uncertainties about the versions actually used in the cited research. Except where explicitly noted, the general character of the measure has remained constant through any revision.

SALT–Systematic Analysis of Language Transcripts

SALT (Miller & Iglesias, 2003–2005) is a Windows®-based computer program that analyzes transcripts of conversations, narratives, and other written texts. The many references to SALT throughout this book reflect my preference for, and experience with, this program. My goal when I talk about SALT, however, is not to promote that program per se, but to share my strong belief in the value of descriptive linguistic analysis for clinical planning. SALT is my tool of choice but you may want to find and use other programs.

I have used SALT ever since the mid-1980s, and find it to be remarkably useful and user-friendly. Judging from my experience in the classroom, if you are relatively comfortable with a computer, you can achieve a good degree of competence with this program in one to two hours. If you are not familiar with SALT, use the website case studies to see its capabilities (www.languageanalysislab.com).

Objectively speaking, SALT is a rather "dumb" concordance program that can only look for specified words (or strings of symbols) and count them. Author Jon Miller and programmer Ann Nockerts, at the University of Wisconsin–Madison, have done an excellent job of making this single function really productive. There are preprogrammed analyses that focus on aspects of syntax, vocabulary, morphology, sentence formulation, and discourse. The results from these preprogrammed search routines can be treated either descriptively or normatively. For example, SALT will calculate the mean length of utterance (MLU) for a language sample either in words or in morphemes, and can also provide a z-score for that MLU indicating how far it lies from the mean MLU earned by children in an age-matched reference group. Similar comparisons can be made for Number of Different Words, Percentage Obligatory Use of Bound Morphemes, Percentage of Utterances that are Question Responses, Percentage of Utterances at Different Lengths that contain false starts, and many other such variables. SALT also allows the user to custom code utterances and will list all of the sentences containing specified forms. The latest version is designed to accept new databases, making it possible to create local norms or work in languages other than English.

Finally, I might add that SALT is a nonprofit venture, and all proceeds are plowed back into program development and support services. The Help screens are excellent and Ms. Nockerts herself is available to provide assistance by phone when all else fails.

Alternate Learning Activities and Discussion Questions

The learning activities at the end of each essay were designed for speech-language pathologists and other child language specialists with clinical or research experience. Graduate students in advanced courses might also have sufficient background to pursue these tasks, but students in introductory courses would find them difficult. Preliminary field testing and questionnaire data helped me to identify a subset of essays as being particularly useful in introductory courses dealing with developmental language disorder. To assist instructors of those courses, Appendix E contains an alternate set of learning activities for these essays. The appendix also repeats activities that were unchanged so that the reader does not need to flip back and forth between lists. The discussion questions for the essays were less biased toward experience, inviting change in only two instances. These new questions are listed at the end of the appendix.

Alternate Learning Activities

Essay 1

1. Review the list of factors and evidence in this essay and think about the implications of this material for parent-child interaction. Create a five-point sheet of advice to parents.

Essay 2

1. Observe one session of direct language intervention with an individual child. Make a list of all of the techniques, procedures, or strategies that are used during the session. Write them in the way needed for preparing an evidence-based practice review.

2. Here are reports of two research studies on similar topics, one with a single-subject design and one with a group design. Read the two articles and write a one-page analysis comparing the strengths and weaknesses of these designs.

   Ellis Weismer, S. E., & Murray-Branch, J. (1989). Modeling versus modeling plus evoked production training: A comparison of two language intervention methods. Journal of Speech and Hearing Disorders, 54(2), 269–281.

Nelson, K. E., Camarata, S. M., Welsh, J., Butkovsky, L., & Camarata, M. (1996). Effects of imitative and conversational recasting treatment on the acquisition of grammar in children with specific language impairment and younger language–normal children. Journal of Speech and Hearing Research, 39, 850–859.

Essay 3

1. Here are two additional dimensions of therapy planning that have barely been investigated. Choose one and do a cost-benefit analysis (i.e., for each position, list the potential benefits and costs, then decide which one is better). You may place higher value on some costs or benefits than on others. Present your analysis as an outline with a concluding paragraph explaining your decision.

   • Criteria for goal completion 40 percent versus 85 percent. For each criterion level, consider cost and benefit if you do or do not use it and it is truly the best way versus if you do or do not use it and it is actually not the best way.

   • Use versus non-use of total communication (i.e., sign + speech) with hearing children. Consider cost and benefits if you assume that this practice will enhance oral language and in fact it is a hindrance versus if you do not make this assumption and hence do not use the technique but in fact it would have helped.

Essay 6

1. There now is a known genetic etiology for Down syndrome. Spend one hour on the Web and attempt to identify one or more treatment strategies that have resulted directly from this scientific advance.

Essay 7

1. Identify a child who seems to have a great number of false starts, self-corrections, pauses, and unfinished utterances. Tape a short language sample. On a sheet of paper, write a column of utterance numbers. Then, as you listen to the tape without transcribing it, count and write down the number of morphemes in each utterance. Listen to the tape one more time and rate each utterance for severity of disruption, on a 1–5 scale. For each of the longer utterances, also note whether the utterance is syntactically complex (2+ clauses, embedded sentence, etc.). Now look at the resulting data. Do the most disrupted utterances tend to be longer? Do disrupted sentences involve sentence complexity? (Your

instructor will assist you in obtaining the tape needed for this exercise if you do not have access to a clinic.)

Essay 8

1. In this essay, I argue that we can give children better tools for organizing information, but cannot improve their memory processes directly. What about all those memory improvement courses? Google "memory improvement" and you will find hundreds of hits—books, drugs, nutrition, software, strategies and yes, courses guaranteed to improve your memory. Spend an hour surfing this motley list. What sorts of strategies are being promoted? Are they usable in therapy with children? Why or why not? Write a one page analysis.

2. Would you expect working memory spans to be the same for visual and auditory-verbal tasks? Conduct some quick tests among yourselves right now using digits, object names, pictures, and gestures. Can you remember the same number of items for each sort of stimulus? Why or why not? Write a brief description of your tasks and the outcomes, with some speculative explanations.

Essay 10

1. The fact that academic, language, and social problems are seen in children with SLI even after they learn to talk, could reflect (1) the effect of some third factor such as processing capacity on both language and other areas of learning, and/or (2) the effects of poor language proficiency on other areas of learning. What sort of evidence would support one or the other of these views? Draw up a "Research to Watch For" list. Add to your list periodically as new issues catch your attention.

Essay 11

1. Check the test section of your departmental or university library to locate any tests of spoken paragraph comprehension or story comprehension (e.g., Gray's Oral Paragraphs, Test of Narrative Language, The Listening Test). For the tests you find, look at the comprehension questions and categorize them into the question types used by Norbury and Bishop. If some question types are not included, write some. Place a brief summary of this activity in the test box so other students can benefit when they interpret the test results.

Essay 12

1. Ask a faculty member in audiology or an audiologist in your community to describe a typical CAPD diagnostic test battery – in detail. If possible, take some portion of the tests yourself and/or discuss how each one contributes to the diagnostic decision. Use this information to list the tasks used in a CAPD assessment and indicate whether they seem to require language, selective attention, and/or working memory.

Essay 13

1. Use the Internet to find out more about the tasks used in the FFW and LLS programs. What do they have in common that could account for the improvement seen with both sets of materials? Gillam argues that both of them promoted selective attention. How?

2. Go to the website for Scientific Learning, the company that markets FFW. What are the strengths and weaknesses of the materials that are presented to demonstrate the value of this program? Rate the level of evidence (see Essay 2) in the research that is cited. (This would be a good group project since there is quite a list of studies to find and evaluate.)

Essay 14

1. Interview a school psychologist, principal, or special education director to find out how your local school district makes use of the traditional diagnostic labels. Are there special programs or resources available for children diagnosed with autism, a learning disability, or other disability?

Essay 15

1. Choose one diagnostic category (e.g., autism, learning disability, SLI, developmental delay) and search the Internet to find information about its speech and language correlates. Spend one hour on this task. Start by going to the website ratings site at Tufts University (www.cfw.tufts.edu) and read their criteria for evaluating online information. When you have finished, make a list of five important things that parents should keep in mind when they consult Internet resources. Prepare a handout.

Essay 16

1. Use The Chart (see pages 123–124) to analyze a language sample (with assistance from SALT, if available). After you have noted particular forms that are

present versus absent or inconsistent, make a list of questions that remain to be answered and create probe tasks that would provide the necessary data.

Essay 17

1. Create a list of three to five ways that you can try to elicit a language form that seems to be missing from the child's repertoire. Each of the steps should provide a further increment of support for use of the language form. Make your assessment sheet generic, so you can use it with any child and any grammatical form that you want to explore during an assessment session. If possible, try out your dynamic assessment scheme with a child (either typically developing or not), focusing on a form that is difficult for the child.

Essay 18

1. Imagine a situation in which you were forced to practice without using any tests at all. Write a one-page essay on what you could and could no longer do.

Essay 20

1. Children are more likely to tell good stories when (1) the number of episodes is manageable; (2) there is some degree of visual support; (3) the scripts are familiar; and (4) the language forms, both lexical and syntactic, are well-known. Write several pairs of stories in which the two members of the pair differ primarily in one of these features. For example, one story has four episodes and the other one only three episodes; or one story is about lunch at McDonalds, and the other story is about changing a flat tire.

Essay 21

1. Write a one-paragraph summary of the FFF framework to explain this approach to special educators and other professionals.

Essay 22

1. Identify a child in your clinic who seems disinterested in or perhaps even resistant to therapy. Make every effort to find out what that child's primary interests are. Ask the child, child's friends, family, or teacher what the child really likes. Observe the child at play if possible. Now, in consultation with the SLP, plan a lesson that incorporates these interests in every possible way. Observe the lesson. Do you see any changes in the child's involvement in the learning tasks? If you lack access to a clinic, invent a child. Then take an activity you have used or observed previously and adapt it to fit this child's

interests. While you're on a roll, adapt the activity for a second child with still different interests. Write a one-page description of the activities and the way that they may or did motivate this child.

Essay 23

1. Make a videotape of yourself interacting with a young child either (a) in a play-based therapy session (preschoolers) or (b) in an unstructured conversation (school age children). If you do not have access to a clinic, do the same with a normally developing child. For the first half of the tape, try to synchronize your activity to the child's activity, i.e. follow the child's lead either verbally or non-verbally. For the second half of the tape, stop trying to follow the child's lead and take more initiative. View the tape. Does the child's behavior change from the first to the second part of the session? How successful were you in monitoring your own turns?

Essay 25

1. Go to a children's bookstore or public library and look for a storybook that you could alter to create focus on a particular language form. Purchase or borrow the book, then get creative and rewrite the text. Think about the mechanics a bit. I typed the new text on my computer, spacing it so I could tape the sheets right over the existing text. That way I can remove them and use the story again in a different fashion. Perhaps you can think of a better system.

Essay 30

1. Choose a nursery rhyme that you do not already know. Ask a friend to tape-record the rhyme, reading with interesting intonation at a comfortable rate. Use this tape to learn the rhyme yourself. How many times do you need to hear it before you can repeat it all yourself? What sorts of errors do you make? What sorts of memory strategies do you use? Does it help to recite the rhyme along with the tape? After you finally succeed in reciting the rhyme, can you remember it five hours later? Two days later?

Essay 31

1. The following eight verbs are normally learned by two- to three-year-olds: *do, drink, drop, go, pretend, push, run, think*. Make a chart and rate each verb 1, 2, or 3 for each of the following characteristics: meaning complexity, predictable perceptual correlates, conceptual availability, and input frequency. A rating of 1 would indicate the easier end of the continuum, (i.e., meaning is simple, there

are reliable perceptual correlates, the necessary concepts are available early, or the word is heard frequently).

When thinking about meaning complexity, think about factors such as whether the verb is causal, how many NPs it requires, or whether it implies an embedded complement sentence. Go with your instinct. It might be easiest to award the 1s and the 3s first, then give the remaining items, if any, a 2.

Add up the four ratings for each word to get a total score. On the basis of these totals, predict the order of acquisition for these words. Low scores should indicate words to be learned first. Now compare your predictions to the real-world facts, as listed at the end of Essay 33 on page 248. Did your predictions pan out? If not, why? Are there other factors we haven't included in the list, or some other explanation for the discrepancies?

Essay 32

1. Go to the norms for the MacArthur-Bates Communicative Development Inventory (www.sci.sdsu.edu/cdi). Ask to see the data for action words at 30 months, in order of frequency. This will give you a list of about 100 verbs that are produced by almost all normally developing children at age 30 months. Print out the list. For each verb, decide which type of meaning it expresses: telic or atelic (or don't know).

2. Take a language sample you have already transcribed, go through it and make a list of all the verbs that the child uses, along with their tense form (e.g., progressive *-ing* or past tense *-ed* and irregulars).(If you have access to the SALT program, this is easily done by asking for a list of all the bound morphemes along with the word roots on which they appear. Otherwise you could use your word processor to find the tense forms, or just scan for verbs by eye). Is there an even distribution of tense forms for telic and atelic verbs? Does the same verb get used with both inflections, or just one?

Essay 35

1. Choose a culture group from among those in your area. Arrange for a consultation session with a member of that community. This could be a parent, a teacher's aide, a daycare worker, or a staff member in the community center. Talk with this person about the values and practices that are typical of families in the culture, especially regarding child rearing and talk to children. Use van Kleeck (1994) to guide your formulation of questions or of an interview protocol.

It is very likely that your consultant will already have thought about cultural differences and will appreciate the opportunity to share his or her views.

Essay 36

1. Put yourself in the shoes of a child learning L2. Invite someone you know who speaks another language, preferably non-Western, to serve as your language model and informant. Invite some classmates over for a two-hour session in which you all attempt to learn this new language. The rule is that your informant cannot speak or respond to English. All exchanges with him or her must be in the new language. Bring props like old clothes and household goods. Divide into teams and plan some sort of interaction. For example, hold up objects and look quizzical, make objects do their typical things while the informant describes your actions, or invent small role-playing vignettes. At the end of an hour or so, tell your informant that he or she can now speak English, and discuss whatever hypotheses you have developed about how the language is organized. Were you on the right track? Did your first language influence your interpretations? Also, explore any communication breakdowns that may have occurred, trying to figure out what went wrong. Loosen up and have fun. I guarantee you will learn something useful about language learning and bilingualism.

NOTE: Before you begin, be sure to ask your informant to (1) ignore pronunciation as much as is possible, (2) speak to you in a simple fashion, as to a young child, and (3) be as helpful as possible—but no English.

Essay 38

1. Collect two language samples from one child, using two different sets of play materials: (1) construction toys (e.g., blocks and cars for boys, art collages or blocks for girls) and (2) role playing toys (e.g., superheros for boys, family dolls for girls). If possible, have a colleague, assistant, or family member actually interact with the child—someone who hasn't read this essay. Analyze and compare the two samples. What is different and what is the same? Look at features such as MLU, speech act functions, syntactic complexity, and turn length.

Alternate Questions for Discussion and Thought

Essay 20

1. If the script is a framework for understanding the general nature of the events in a story, what sort of framework is the story grammar? What does it organize? What are its units?

2. This essay argues that story content/organization and grammaticality can trade off in a limited capacity system and, further, that this tradeoff results from the child's own focus. That is, in some circumstances, a child will choose to be grammatical even if this results in a poor story. Does this possibility make sense? Can you think of a different way to explain the trade-off data?

3. Robertson and Ellis Weismer (1997) report a study in which children with SLI improved their ability to tell scripts for playing in the doll corner following time spent playing with a normally developing peer. Can we assume from this fact that these children also told better stories about doll corner types of events? Why and/or why not?

Essay 23

1. What are the options when you need to establish a collaborative relationship with someone (e.g., teacher, occupational therapist, parent) who holds theoretical views that conflict with your own?

2. This essay argues that every program is comprised of two or more components that can be unbundled and manipulated. What do you see as the possible advantages and disadvantages of pulling programs apart in this fashion? Is your answer different for programs with and without proven efficacy?

3. This essay describes an important change in my understanding of the therapy process. What constitutes responsible, ethical practice? If there is a preferred procedure (or a disproven one), and it is not used (or is used) because the SLP is unaware of the pertinent facts, what should the SLP do when she or he later learns of them?

Glossary

NOTE: The following terms and definitions are meant only to assist the reader in understanding the ideas presented in this book, and are not comprehensive.

ABA. Applied Behavioral Analysis; an approach to intervention developed by Ivar Lovaas that is widely used for children diagnosed with autism spectrum disorder. The approach draws on Skinnerian Behaviorism, is highly structured and teacher directed, presents decontextualized language, and uses extrinsic rewards.

AMERICAN SPEECH-LANGUAGE-HEARING ASSOCIATION (ASHA). The professional organization of speech-language pathologists and audiologists in the United States.

ANAPHORIC PRONOUNS. Pronouns that refer back to persons that have been mentioned earlier; in contrast to exophoric pronouns that refer to persons who are physically present in the communication context but haven't yet been mentioned.

ASHA. See American Speech-Language-Hearing Association.

ASYMPTOTIC LEARNING. Learning in a domain with a fixed and limited content; after a period of rapid gain, there is little or nothing left to learn and the learning curve flattens as it approaches the asymptote (i.e., straight line) of total knowledge.

BOTTOM-UP PROCESSING. Information processing that is exclusively data driven. Used to describe mental functions that ascertain and store properties of perceptual events such as frequency. (See also Top-Down Processing.)

COCHRANE COLLABORATION. An international nonprofit and independent organization, dedicated to making up-to-date, accurate information about the effects of healthcare readily available worldwide. It produces and disseminates systematic reviews of healthcare interventions.

COGNITION. Any aspect of mental function, including memory, attention, coordinating and planning, problem solving, world knowledge, and abstract conceptualization. Frequently divided into verbal versus nonverbal cognition, or processing mechanisms versus represented knowledge.

COHESION. A property of narratives or other written and spoken texts that results when language forms such as pronouns, articles, conjunctions, and lexical repetitions are used to explicitly indicate the connections between earlier and later passages.

COHERENCE. A property of narratives or other written and spoken texts that results when the various sections are organized in a logically, causally, and/or temporally satisfying manner.

COMPETENCE. A quality ascribed to persons who have the knowledge and skill required for a given act. Often contrasted with performance.

CONNECTIONISM. A broad perspective on cognitive function and architecture that attempts to explain human development and behavior as resulting from the activation levels, linkages, and inhibitory acts of neural networks.

CONSTRUCTIVISM. A broad perspective on human development that emphasizes the interpreting and organizing activities of the child, and thus treats knowledge as ultimately constructed, rather than transferred or recorded.

COORDINATE BILINGUALISM. The ability to use two or more languages with equal facility.

COUNT NOUN. A noun that can be modified by a numeral and occurs in both singular and plural form. Contrasts with Mass Noun.

DISCOURSE. An organized unit of language larger than the utterance; may be multispeaker and collaborative as in a conversation, or single-speaker as in a narrative or a lecture.

DYNAMIC ASSESSMENT. An approach to language (or cognitive) assessment that looks at the way performance changes over time, with and without adult assistance, in contrast to the more traditional practice of measuring a given capability at a single point in time. The time interval may span minutes or months.

DUAL-TASK EXPERIMENT. An experiment that requires performance of two simultaneous tasks; success on the secondary task indicates how much processing capacity was used up by the primary task.

ELICITED IMITATION. A procedure used in language assessment or therapy in which the child is told to repeat the sound, word, or utterance spoken by the interventionist.

EVIDENCE-BASED PRACTICE. The process of evaluating bodies of research in a systematic fashion to ascertain best practice.

EVOKED PRODUCTION. A procedure used in language assessment or therapy in which a communicative context is set up that will invite, if not compel, the use of a particular language form or class of forms.

Exophoric Pronouns. Pronouns that refer to persons who are physically present in the communication context but haven't yet been mentioned; in contrast to anaphoric pronouns that refer back to persons that have been mentioned earlier.

Experimental Research Design. Design in which the researcher assigns subjects to groups, there is at least one control group, and the researcher controls the independent variables including the treatment. The strongest versions will also have randomized assignment to groups.

Fast ForWord®. A controversial family of computer-based, individualized instructional programs focused on language comprehension, auditory perception, and reading. The language programs make use of acoustically altered speech that is ultimately intended to improve the temporal processing capabilities of the user.

Fast Mapping. The first stage of word learning in which a child enters a new word into his/her lexicon after one or two hearings; initial meanings are limited and the phonological rendering may be imperfect.

Focused Modeling. A procedure used in language therapy in which the therapist provides an unusually large number of examples of the form to be learned within a set time frame.

Infralogical. In Piagetian theory, a category of knowledge that is organized around spatial, temporal, or causal operations (e.g., *become, be part of, cause*) rather than logical operations (e.g., *be instance of, and, if*). Used more generally to refer to any nonlogical thought.

Isomorphic. Having point-to-point correspondence with another entity; more generally, having the same shape or structure.

LA. Language age. Used to describe the level of a child's language knowledge and use by equating it to the average performance of children at some specific age.

Language Sample Analysis (LSA). An approach to language assessment which uses the child's spontaneously produced speech rather than responses to test items. Once collected, the language sample can be analyzed linguistically and the child's language competence inferred from this analysis. Spontaneous speech data can also be treated in a normative fashion using standardized scoring systems (DSS, IPSyn) or SALT (see Appendixes C and D).

Late Talker. A diagnostic or research category that refers to children age 24 months or younger whose language behavior falls below the 10th percentile.

LIMITED-CAPACITY SYSTEM. A system that can perform only a finite number of operations at any given time, such as the human mind and its cognitive functions.

LSA. See Language Sample Analysis.

MA. Mental age. Used to describe the general level of a child's intellectual development by equating it to the average performance of children at some specific age.

MASTERY LEARNING. The later stages of learning a word or grammatical pattern, during which deployment of the form becomes more efficient and automatic and/or the form's meanings and uses are enriched.

MAZE. In the SALT program, a maze is any material within an utterance that does not contribute to the final sentence product, e.g., false starts, self-repetitions, filled pauses, reformulations. This material is set off in parentheses and does not contribute to the MLU calculation.

MEAN LENGTH OF UTTERANCE (MLU). The average length of utterances in a language sample, in words or morphemes; correlates with age and with other aspects of language knowledge and provides a general index of language proficiency.

META-ANALYSIS. A statistical procedure in which the findings from a number of studies are combined into one grand test of the size and significance of an effect; used widely in evidence-based practice reviews to evaluate effects of treatment.

MLU. See Mean Length of Utterance.

NARRATIVE. A cover term for a range of single-speaker texts, including stories, and the relating of personal events; can be recalled, retold, or newly created; generally consists of a series of connected events caused or experienced by participants.

NONCE WORD/VERB. A term referring to nonstandard or nonsensical words. Nonce words usually conform to the phonotactic rules of the language and can be thought of as potential words.

NP. Noun phrase.

PERFORMANCE. The actual doing of something, which may or may not make effective use of all of the doers capabilities; often contrasted with competence. Example: a given utterance may not include all of the grammatical forms that a child has demonstrated knowledge of on other occasions.

PDD. Pervasive developmental disorder; a generic term for a group of disorders that involve social interaction; verbal and nonverbal communication; and stereotypic behaviors.

PRAGMATICS. Language use as influenced by the social, topical, intentional, physical, and linguistic context; effective communication requires the selection of the right forms for particular moments, listeners, and communicative intents.

PROBE TASK. A language task created by a therapist or educator to assess a child's knowledge of a particular form; used to confirm or disconfirm the initial conclusions drawn from a language sample or other observation.

PROCESSING CAPACITY. The amount of work that is doable in a unit of time.

QUASI-EXPERIMENTAL RESEARCH DESIGN. Design in which one or more of the independent variables cannot be controlled by the researcher (e.g., a pre-existing trait) and/or the treatment/experience is already underway; otherwise similar to experimental design. (Definitions of this design are quite diverse, but this one is representative.)

SALT. See Systematic Analysis of Language Transcripts.

SCRIPT. A mental outline of the general types and sequences of subevents that are likely to occur in a particular event context, such as going to the movies, eating out, visiting the doctor's office.

SD. See Standard Deviation.

SINGLE-SUBJECT RESEARCH DESIGN. Design in which each subject serves as his or her own control; often uses multiple baseline measurements (e.g., the learning target and an untreated behavior); may be more than one subject in the study.

SLI. See Specific Language Impairment.

SLP. See Speech-Language Pathologist.

SPECIFIC LANGUAGE IMPAIRMENT (SLI). A developmental condition in which language skills appear to be developing at a notably slower rate than other aspects of mind and body. Occurs in the absence of sensory, motor, or affective disorder, and does not imply a general mental retardation. Formerly known as developmental aphasia, developmental language disorder, and dysphasia.

Thinking About Child Language

SPEECH-LANGUAGE PATHOLOGIST (SLP). A professional who facilitates the acquisition or recovery of verbal communication skills. This rather unwieldy professional title must have been invented by a committee but does reflect a scope of practice that has widened from a focus on speech sounds to the current inclusion of virtually all aspects of language learning and use. The title also acknowledges the biological bases of human language and its linkage to health. The acronym is now commonly used in lieu of the full title—and is pronounced "S-L-P."

STANDARD DEVIATION *(SD).* A statistical measure that provides information about the range and distribution of scores around the Mean. The interval of Mean +/-1 *SD* includes about 67 percent of the scores. A large *SD* signifies greater variability.

STORY GRAMMAR. A culture-specific mental outline that specifies the elements of a good story and the order in which they should occur.

SYSTEMATIC ANALYSIS OF LANGUAGE TRANSCRIPTS (SALT). See Appendix D.

TOP-DOWN PROCESSING. Information processing that makes use of prior knowledge to anticipate, organize, and interpret new data.

TOTAL COMMUNICATION. A procedure borrowed from educators of the deaf in which child-directed speech is accompanied by signs and/or natural gesture. The procedure usually makes use of hybrid systems such as Signed English, which takes basic signs from American Sign Language but presents them in the order dictated by spoken English and without any of the other grammatical features of the signed language.

UNIVERSAL GRAMMAR. A psychological construct proposed by theorists as an explanation for the rapid, early, and apparently effortless acquisition of language by young children. Broadly defined, universal grammar is a genetically provided representation of all of the grammatical options occurring in human language, leaving the child only the task of deciding which ones are true of the language she or he experiences.

ZONE OF PROXIMAL DEVELOPMENT. A term introduced by Vygotsky to refer to the disparity between what the chid can do independently and what he or she can do with guidance and support of those with more experience. Similar to what other theorists have called the *competence–performance gap,* or the *bandwidth of competence.*

References

Akhtar, N., Carpenter, M., & Tomasello, M. (1996). The role of discourse novelty in children's early word learning. *Child Development, 67,* 635–645.

American Psychiatric Association. (1994). *Diagnostic and statistical manual of mental disorders* (4th ed.). Washington, DC: Author.

American Speech-Language-Hearing Association. (2005a). *(Central) auditory processing disorders: The role of the audiologist.* Retrieved June, 2005, from http://www.asha.org/members/deskref-journals

American Speech-Language-Hearing Association. (2005b). *Evidence-based practice in communication disorders* [Position Statement]. Retrieved September, 2005, from http://asha.org/members/deskrefjournals/deskref/default

Baddeley, A. (1986). *Working memory.* Oxford: Oxford University Press.

Ball, C., Sackett, D., Phillips, B., Haynes, B., Straus, S., & Dawes, M. (2001, February). *Oxford Centre for Evidence-Based Medicine levels of evidence.* Retrieved September, 2005, from www.cebm.net

Bartlett, C., Flax, J., Logue, M., Vieland, V., Bassett, A., Tallal, P., et al. (2002). A major susceptibility locus for specific language impairment is located on 13q21. *American Journal of Human Genetics, 71,* 45–55.

Bates, E. (1979). *The emergence of symbols.* New York: Academic Press.

Bates, E., & Goodman, J. (1997). On the inseparability of grammar and the lexicon. *Language and Cognitive Processes, 12,* 507–584.

Bates, E., & MacWhinney, B. (1982). Functionalist approaches to grammar. In E. Wanner & L. Gleitman (Eds.), *Language acquisition: The state of the art* (pp. 273–318). New York: Cambridge University Press.

Behrend, D., Harris, L. L., & Cartwright, K. (1995). Morphological cues to verb meaning: Verb inflections and the initial mapping of verb meanings. *Journal of Child Language, 22,* 89–106.

Beitchman, J., Wilson, B., Johnson, C., Atkinson, L., Young, A., Adlaf, E., et al. (2001). Fourteen year follow-up of speech/language impaired and control children: Psychiatric outcome. *Journal of the American Academy of Child and Adolescent Psychiatry, 40*(1), 75–82.

Bialystok, E., & Martin, M. (2004). Attention and inhibition in bilingual children. *Developmental Science, 7,* 325–339.

Bialystok, E., Martin, M., & Viswanathan, Z. (in press). Bilingualism across the lifespan: The rise and fall of inhibitory control. *International Journal of Bilingualism.*

Bishop, D., Carlyon, R., Deeks, J., & Bishop, S. (1999). Auditory temporal processing impairment: Neither necessary nor sufficient for causing language impairment in children. *Journal of Speech, Language, and Hearing Research, 42*, 1295–1310.

Bishop, D., & Edmundson, A. (1987). Language impaired 4 year olds: Distinguishing transient from persistent impairment. *Journal of Speech and Hearing Disorders, 52*, 156–173.

Bishop, D., North, T., & Donlan, C. (1995). Genetic basis of specific language impairment: Evidence from a twin study. *Developmental Medicine and Child Neurology, 37*, 56–71.

Bock, J. K. (1982). Towards a cognitive psychology of syntax: Information processing contributions to sentence formulation. *Psychological Review, 89*, 1–47.

Bock, K., & Levelt, W. (1994). Language production: Grammatical encoding. In M. A. Gernsbacher (Ed.), *Handbook of psycholinguistics* (pp. 945–984). San Diego: Academic Press.

Boswell, S. (2005, March 22). Prevention model takes off in schools. *The ASHA Leader, 1*, 20–21.

Botting, N., Faragher, B., Simkin, Z., Knox, E., & Conti-Ramsden, G. (2001). Predicting pathways of specific language impairment: What differentiates good and poor outcomes? *Journal of Child Psychology and Psychiatry and Allied Disciplines, 42*, 1013–1020.

Brown, A., & Reeve, R. (1987). Bandwidths of competence: The role of supportive contexts in learning and development. In L. Liben (Ed.), *Development and learning: Conflict or congruence* (pp. 173–223). Hillsdale, NJ: Erlbaum.

Brown, R. (1973). *A first language: The early stages*. Cambridge, MA: Harvard University Press.

Bryant, P., Bradley, L., Maclean, M., & Crossland, J. (1989). Nursery rhymes, phonological skills, and reading. *Journal of Child Language, 16*, 407–418.

Buros Institute. (1938–2005). *Mental measurements yearbook*. Highland Park, NJ: Gryphon Press.

Caesar, L. (2005, June). *SLPs' use of alternative language assessment procedures with bilingual children*. Paper presented at the Symposium on Research in Child Language Disorders, Madison, WI.

Carr, L., & Johnston, J. (2001). Morphological cues to verb meaning. *Applied Psycholinguistics, 22*, 601–618.

Catts, H., Chermak, G., Craig, C., Johnston, J., Keith, R., Musiek, F., et al. (1996). Central auditory processing: Current status of research and implications for clinical practice. *American Journal of Audiology, 5*, 41–54.

Catts, H., Fey, M., & Zhang, X. (2001). Estimating the risk of future reading difficulties in kindergarten children: A research-based model and its clinical implementation. *Language, Speech, and Hearing Services in Schools 32*, 38–50.

Catts, H., Fey, M., Zhang, X., & Tomblin, B. (1999). Language basis of reading and reading disabilities: Evidence from a longitudinal investigation. *Scientific Studies of Reading, 3*(4), 331–361.

Chao, R. (1995). Beyond parental control and authoritarian parenting style: Understanding Chinese parenting through the cultural notion of training. *Child Development, 65,* 111–119.

Charman, T., Baron-Cohen, S., Swettenham, J., Baird, G., Drew, A., & Cox, A. (2003). Predicting language outcome in infants with autism and pervasive developmental disorder. *International Journal of Language and Communication Disorders, 38,* 265–285.

Chaudhary, N. (1999). Language socialization: Patterns of caregiver speech to young children. In T. S. Saraswathi (Ed.), *Culture, socialization, and human development: Theory, research, and applications in India* (pp. 145–166). Thousand Oaks, CA: Sage.

Chermak, G., Hall, J., & Musiek, F. (1999). Differential diagnosis and management of central auditory processing disorder and attention deficit hyperactivity disorder. *Journal of the American Academy of Audiology, 10,* 289–303.

Chomsky, N. (1959). A review of B. F. Skinner's *Verbal Behavior. Language, 35,* 26–58.

Clark, E. (1993). *The lexicon in acquisition.* Cambridge, UK: Cambridge University Press.

Clark, H., & Fox Tree, J. (2002). Using uh and um in spontaneous speaking. *Cognition, 84,* 73–111.

Cloud, J. (2003). How we get labeled. *Time, 161*(3), 102–105.

Cole, K., & Dale, P. (1986). Direct language instruction and interactive language instruction with language delayed preschool children: A comparison study. *Journal of Speech and Hearing Research, 29,* 206–217.

Colozzo, P., Curan, M., Garcia, R., Gillam, R., & Johnston, J. (2006). *Grammatical error as an index of capacity limitations in narrative.* Manuscript submitted for publication. University of British Columbia, Vancouver.

Condouris, K., Meyer, C., & Tager-Flusberg, H. (2003). The relationship between standardized measures of language and measures of spontaneous speech in children with autism. *American Journal of Speech Language Pathology, 12,* 349–358.

Connell, P., & Stone, A. (1992). Morpheme learning of children with specific language impairment under controlled instructional conditions. *Journal of Speech, Language, and Hearing Research, 35,* 844–852.

Connor, C., Morrison, F., & Katch, L. (2004). Beyond the reading wars: Exploring the effect of child-instruction interactions on growth in early reading. *Scientific Studies of Reading, 8,* 305–336.

Crawford, J. (1997). *Opinion polls on official english.* Retrieved June, 2005, from Language Policy Web Site & Emporium, http://ourworld.compuserve.com/homepages/JWCRAWFORD/can-poll.htm

Crawford, J. (2002). *Census 2000: A guide for the perplexed*. Retrieved June, 2005, from Language Policy Web Site and Emporium, http://ourworld.compuserve.com/homepages/JWCRAW-FORD/census02.htm

Crystal, D., Fletcher, P., & Garman, M. (1976). *Grammatical analysis of language ability*. London: Edward Arnold.

Culatta, B., & Horn, D. (1982). A program for achieving generalization of grammatical rules to spontaneous discourse. *Journal of Speech and Hearing Disorders, 47*, 174–180.

Curan, M., Colozzo, P., & Johnston, J. (2004, October). *The test of narrative language: Form vs. content*. Paper presented at the annual meeting of the British Columbia Association of Speech Language Pathologists and Audiologists, Kelowna, BC.

Dale, P., & Fenson, L. (1996). Lexical development norms in young children. *Behavioral research Methods, Instruments, and Computers, 28*, 25–127. Retrieved November 27, 2005, from www.sci.sdsu.edu/cdi/lexical_e.htm

Dale, P., Simonoff, E., Bishop, D., Eley, T., Oliver, B., Price, T., et al. (1998). Genetic influence on language delay in two-year-old children. *Nature Neuroscience, 1*, 324–328.

Deci, E., Koestner, R., & Ryan, R. (1999). A meta-analytic review of experiments examining the effects of extrinsic rewards on intrinsic motivation. *Psychological Bulletin, 125*, 627–668.

De Fosse, L., Hodge, S., Makris, N., Kennedy, D., Caviness, V., McGrath, L., et al. (2004). Language association cortex asymmetry in autism and specific language impairment. *Annals of Neurology, 56*, 757–766.

Delprato, D. (2001). Comparisons of discrete trial and normalized behavioral language intervention. *Journal of Autism and Developmental Disorders, 31*, 315–325.

deVilliers, P., & deVilliers, J. (1972). Early judgments of semantic and syntactic acceptability by children. *Journal of Psycholinguistic Research, 1*, 299–310.

Doherty, J. (1985). The effects of sign characteristics on sign acquisition and retention: An integrative review of the literature. *AAC: Augmentative and Alternative Communication, 1*, 108–121.

Dollaghan, C. (2004, April 13). Evidence-based practice: Myths and realities. *The ASHA Leader, 12*, 4–5.

Donlan, C. (2003). *Number talk*. Retrieved June, 2005, from www.ucl.ac.uk/HCS/research/numbertalkproject.htm

Drew, A., Baird, G., & Baron-Cohen, S. (2002). A pilot randomized control trial of a parent training intervention for preschool children with autism: Preliminary findings and methodological challenges. *European Child and Adolescent Psychiatry, 11*, 266–272.

Eisenberg, S., Fersko, T., & Lundgren, C. (2001). The use of MLU for identifying language impairment in preschool children: A review. *American Journal of Speech-Language Pathology, 10*, 323–342.

References

Ellis, J., Mulligan, I., Rowe, J., & Sackett, D. (1995). Inpatient general medicine is evidence based. *Lancet, 346,* 407–410.

Ellis Weismer, S. (1990–1991). Theory and practice: A principled approach to treatment of young children with specific language disorders. *National Student Speech Language Hearing Association Journal, 18,* 76–86.

Ellis Weismer, S. (1996). Capacity limitations in working memory: The impact on lexical and morphological learning by children with language impairment. *Topics in Language Disorders, 17,* 33–44.

Ellis Weismer, S., & Hesketh, L. (1993). The influence of prosodic and gestural cues on novel word acquisition by children with specific language impairment. *Journal of Speech and Hearing Research, 36,* 1013–1025.

Ellis Weismer, S., & Murray-Branch, J. (1989). Modeling versus modeling plus evoked production training: A comparison of two language intervention methods. *Journal of Speech and Hearing Disorders, 54,* 269–281.

Ellis Weismer, S., & Thordardottir, E. (2002). Cognition and language. In P. Accardo, B. Rogers, & A. Capute (Eds.), *Disorders of language development* (pp. 21–37). Timonium, MD: York Press.

Elman, J., Bates, E., Johnson, M., Karmiloff-Smith, A., Parisi, D., & Plunkett, K. (1996). *Rethinking innateness: A connectionist perspective on development.* Cambridge, MA: MIT Press.

Fawcett, S. (2003). *A comparison of two approaches to assessing language change in children with autism.* Unpublished master's thesis, University of British Columbia, Vancouver, British Columbia, Canada.

Fawcett, S., & Johnston, J. (2003, November). *Assessing language change in children with autism: A comparison of two approaches.* Paper presented at the annual meeting of the American Speech-Language-Hearing Association, Chicago, IL.

Fazio, B. (1994). The counting abilities of children with specific language impairment: A comparison of oral and gestural tasks. *Journal of Speech and Hearing Research, 37,* 358–368.

Fazio, B. (1996). Mathematical abilities of children with specific language impairment: A two year followup. *Journal of Speech and Hearing Research, 42,* 839–849.

Fazio, B. (1997a). Learning a new poem. *Journal of Speech, Language, and Hearing Research, 40,* 1285–1297.

Fazio, B. (1997b). Memory for rote linguistic routines and sensitivity to rhyme. *Applied Psycholinguistics, 18,* 345–372.

Fazio, B. (1999). Arithmetic calculation, short term memory and language performance in children with specific language impairment: A five year follow-up. *Journal of Speech, Language, and Hearing Research, 42,* 420–431.

Fazio, B., Johnston, J. R., & Brandl, L. (1993). Relationship between mental age and vocabulary development among children with mild mental retardation. *American Journal of Mental Retardation, 97,* 541–546.

Fernandez-Fein, S., & Baker, L. (1997). Rhyme and alliteration sensitivity and relevant experiences among preschoolers from diverse backgrounds. *Journal of Literacy Research, 29,* 433–459.

Fey, M. (1986). *Language intervention with young children.* San Diego: College Hill.

Fey, M., Cleave, P., Long, S., & Hughs, D. (1993). Two approaches to the facilitation of grammar in language impaired children: An experimental evaluation. *Journal of Speech and Hearing Research, 36,* 141–157.

Fillmore, L. W. (1996). What happens when languages are lost? An essay on language assimilation and cultural identity. In D. Slobin & J. Gerhardt (Eds.), *Social interaction, social context and language: Essays in honor of Susan Ervin-Tripp* (pp. 435–446). Hillsdale, NJ: Erlbaum.

Fletcher, P. (1992). Subgroups in school age language impaired children. In P. Fletcher & D. Hall (Eds.), *Specific speech and language disorders in children.* London: Whurr.

Freeman, L., & Miller, A. (2001). Norm-referenced, criterion-referenced, and dynamic assessment: What exactly is the point? *Educational Psychology in Practice, 17,* 3–16.

Friedman, P., & Friedman, K. (1980). Accounting for individual differences when comparing the effectiveness of remedial language teaching methods. *Applied Psycholinguistics, 1,* 127–150.

Frome Loeb, D., Stoke, C., & Fey, M. (2001). Language changes associated with Fast ForWord–Language: Evidence from case studies. *American Journal of Speech-Language Pathology, 10,* 216–230.

Garcia, R. (2005). *Linguistic tradeoffs among syntax and semantics in the narrative language of typically developing children and children with specific language impairment.* Unpublished master's thesis, University of Texas, Austin, Texas.

Gardner, H. (1993). *Frames of mind: The theory of multiple intelligences* (10th ed.). New York: Basic Books.

Gaulin, C., & Campbell, T. (1994). Procedure for assessing verbal working memory in normal school age children: Some preliminary data. *Perceptual and Motor Skills, 79,* 55–64.

Gentner, D. (1982). Why nouns are learned before verbs: Linguistic relativity vs. natural partitioning. In S. Kuczaj (Ed.), *Language development: Vol. 2.* (pp. 301–334). Mahwah, NJ: Erlbaum.

Gillam, R. B. (1996). Putting memory to work in language intervention: Implications for practitioners. *Topics in Language Disorders, 18,* 72–79.

Gillam, R. B. (1999). Treatment for temporal processing deficits: Computer-assisted language intervention using Fast ForWord: Theoretical and empirical considerations for clinical decision making. *Language, Speech, and Hearing Services in Schools, 30,* 363–370.

Gillam, R. (2005, June). *A randomized comparison of language intervention programs.* Paper presented at the Symposium on Research in Child Language Disorders, Madison, WI.

Gillam, R., Crofford, J., Gale, M., & Hoffman, L. (2001). Language change following computer-assisted language instruction with Fast ForWord or Laureate Learning Systems software. *American Journal of Speech Language Pathology, 10,* 231–247.

Gillam, R., Frome Loeb, D., & Friel-Patti, S. (2001). Looking back: A summary of five exploratory studies of Fast ForWord. *American Journal of Speech Language Pathology, 10,* 269–273.

Gillette, J., Gleitman, H., Gleitman, L., & Lederer, A. (1999). Human simulations of vocabulary learning. *Cognition, 73,* 135–176.

Gillman, M., Heyman, B., & Swain, J. (2000). What's in a name? The implications of diagnosis for people with learning difficulties and their family carers. *Disability and Society, 15,* 389–409.

Girolametto, L., Pearce, P., & Weitzman, E. (1996). Interactive focused stimulation for toddlers with expressive vocabulary delays. *Journal of Speech, Language, and Hearing Research, 39,* 1274–1283.

Goldstein, H. (2002). Communication intervention for children with autism: A review of treatment efficacy. *Journal of Autism and Developmental Disorders, 32,* 373–396.

Goodwyn, S., & Acredolo, L. (1993). Symbolic gesture vs word: Is there a modality advantage for onset of symbol use? *Child Development, 64,* 688–791.

Goodwyn, S., Acredolo, L., & Brown, C. (2000). Impact of symbolic gesturing on early language development. *Journal of Nonverbal Behavior, 24,* 81–103.

Gutierrez-Clellen, V., Calderon, J., & Ellis Weismer, S. (2004). Verbal working memory in bilingual children. *Journal of Speech, Language, and Hearing Research, 47,* 863–876.

Gutierrez-Clellen, V., & Peña, E. (2001). Dynamic assessment of diverse children: A tutorial. *Language, Speech, and Hearing Services in Schools, 32,* 212–224.

Hamilton, C., Coates, R., & Heffernan, T. (2003). What develops in visuo-spatial working memory development? *European Journal of Cognitive Psychology, 15*(1), 43–69.

Hart, E., & Risley, T. (1995). *Meaningful differences in the everyday experiences of young American children.* Baltimore: Brookes.

Haywood, H. C., Brooks, P., & Burns, S. (1992). *Bright Start: Cognitive curriculum for young children.* New York: Charlesbridge.

Hess, L., & Johnston, J. (1988). Acquisition of back channel responses to adequate messages. *Discourse Processes, 11,* 319–336.

Hoff-Ginsberg, E., & Shatz, M. (1982). Linguistic input and the child's acquisition of language. *Psychological Bulletin, 82,* 3–26.

Holmes, O. W. (1918). Towne v Eisner. *U.S. Reporter, 245*(418), 425.

Hudson, J., & Shapiro, L. (1991). From knowing to telling: The development of scripts, stories, and personal narratives. In A. McCabe & C. Peterson (Eds.), *Developing narrative structure* (pp. 89–136). Hillsdale, NJ: Erlbaum.

Im-Bolter, N. (2003). *Executive processes and mental attention in children with language impairment.* Unpublished doctoral dissertation, York University, Toronto, Canada.

Johnston, J. (1982a). Interpreting the Leiter IQ: Performance profiles of young normal and language disordered children. *Journal of Speech and Hearing Research, 25,* 291–296.

Johnston, J. (1982b). Narratives: A new look at communication problems in older language disordered children. *Language, Speech, and Hearing Services in Schools, 13,* 65–75.

Johnston, J. (1985a). Cognitive prerequisites: The evidence from children learning English. In D. Slobin (Ed.), *The cross-linguistic study of child language acquisition: Vol. 2.* (pp. 961–1004). Hillsdale, NJ: Erlbaum.

Johnston, J. (1985b). Fit, focus, and functionality: An essay on early language intervention. *Child Language Teaching and Therapy, 1*(2), 125–134.

Johnston, J. (1988). Specific language disorders in the child. In N. Lass, L. McReynolds, J. Northern, & D. Yoder (Eds.), *Handbook of speech-language pathology and audiology* (pp. 685–715). Philadelphia: B.C. Decker.

Johnston, J. (1999). Cognitive deficits in specific language impairment: Decision in spite of uncertainty. *Journal of Speech Language Pathology and Audiology, 23,* 65–172.

Johnston, J. (2001). An alternate MLU calculation: Magnitude and variability of effects. *Journal of Speech, Language, and Hearing Research, 44,* 1362–1375.

Johnston, J. (2005). Factors that influence language development. In R. Tremblay, R. Barr, & R. Peters (Eds.), *Encyclopedia on early childhood development* [online]. Montreal: Centre for Excellence for Early Childhood Development; 2005:1–6. Available at www.excellence–earlychildhood.ca/documents/JohnstonANGxp.pdf

Johnston, J., & Ammon, M. (1985c). *The Chart.* Unpublished manuscript.

Johnston J., & Ellis Weismer, S. (1983). Mental rotation abilities in language disordered children. *Journal of Speech and Hearing Research, 26,* 397–403.

Johnston, J., Miller, J. F., Curtiss, S., & Tallal, P. (1993). Conversations with children who are language impaired: Asking questions. *Journal of Speech, Language, and Hearing Research, 36,* 973–978.

Johnston, J., Miller, J., & Tallal, P. (2001). Use of cognitive state predicates by language impaired children. *International Journal of Language and Communication Disorders, 36,* 349–370.

Johnston, J., & Ramstad, V. (1983). Cognitive development in preadolescent language impaired children. *British Journal of Disorders of Communication, 18*, 49–55.

Johnston, J., & Slobin, D. (1979). The development of locative expressions in English, Italian, Serbo-Croation, and Turkish. *Journal of Child Language, 6*, 529–545.

Johnston, J., & Smith, L. (1989). Dimensional thinking in language impaired children. *Journal of Speech and Hearing Research, 32*, 33–38.

Johnston, J., & Welsh, E. (2000). Comprehension of "because" and "so": The role of prior event representation. *First Language, 20*, 291–304.

Johnston, J., & Wong, A. (2002). Cultural differences in beliefs and practices concerning talk to children. *Journal of Speech, Language, and Hearing Research, 45*, 916–926.

Kamhi, A. (1981). Nonlinguistic symbolic and conceptual abilities in language impaired and normally developing children. *Journal of Speech and Hearing Research, 24*, 446–453.

Kamhi, A., Gentry, B., Mauer, D., & Gholson, B. (1990). Analogical learning and transfer in language-impaired children. *Journal of Speech and Hearing Disorders, 55*, 140–148.

Kamhi, A., & Nelson, L. (1988). Early syntactic development. *Topics in Language Development, 8*(2), 42–43.

Kanner, L. (1971). Follow-up study of eleven autistic children originally reported in 1943. *Journal of Autism and Childhood Schizophrenia, 1*, 119–145.

Kay-Raining Bird, E., Cleave, P., Trudeau, N., Thordardottir, E., Sutton, A., & Thorpe, A. (2005). The language abilities of bilingual children with Down Syndrome. *American Journal of Speech-Language Pathology, 14*, 187–199.

Kerr, A., Guildford, S., & Kay-Raining Bird, E. (2003). Standardized language test use: A Canadian survey. *Journal of Speech-Language Pathology and Audiology, 27*, 10–28.

Kester, E., Peña, E., & Gillam, R. (2001). Outcomes of dynamic assessment with culturally and linguistically diverse students: A comparison of three teaching methods within a test-teach-retest framework. *Journal of Cognitive Education and Psychology, 2*, 42–59.

Kidshealth. (2004). *Central auditory processing disorder*. Retrieved June, 2005, from Kidshealth website, section for parents, under Medical conditions of the ear: http://kidshealth.org/parent/

Kjelgaard, M., & Tager-Flusberg, H. (2001). An investigation of language impairment in autism: Implications for genetic subgroups. *Language and Cognitive Processes, 16*, 287–308.

Kritikos, E. (2003). Speech-language pathologists' beliefs about language assessment of bilingual/bicultural individuals. *American Journal of Speech-Language Pathology, 12*, 73–91.

Krowchuk, R. (2005). *English as a second language: Funding and costs*. Retrieved June, 2005, from Vancouver School Board website, ESL Programs, Interoffice Memorandum: http://www.vsb.bc.ca

Thinking About Child Language

Kuhn, D. (1972). Mechanisms of change in the development of cognitive structures. *Child Development, 43,* 833–844.

Kwok, A. (2002, Spring). Family centered service coordination—A paradigm shift in working with children with disabilities. *Rehab Review, 7–9.* Retrieved from www.education.uiowa.edu/rehab/newsletter/Spring202004/newsletter_spring_2004.htm

Lahey, M. (1988). *Language disorders and language development.* New York: McMillan.

Lao-Tzu. (520). *Chapter 32, Sentence #4 (Stephen Mitchell, Trans.).* Retrieved July 7, 2005, from Tao Teh Ching Comparison Project, http://wayist.org

Leadholm, B., & Miller, J. (1992). *Language sample analysis guide.* Madison, WI: Wisconsin Department of Public Instruction.

Leaper, C., & Smith, T. (2004). A meta-analytic view of gender variations in children's language use: Talkativeness, affiliative speech and assertive speech. *Developmental Psychology, 40,* 993–1027.

Leonard, L. (1975). The role of non-linguistic stimuli and semantic relations in children's acquisition of grammatical utterances. *Journal of Experimental Child Psychology, 19,* 346–357.

Leonard, L. (1992). The use of morphology by children with specific language impairment: Evidence from three languages. In R. Chapman (Ed.), *Processes in language acquisition and disorders* (pp. 186–201). St. Louis: Mosby–Yearbook.

Leonard, L. (1998). *Children with specific language impairment.* Cambridge, MA: MIT Press.

Lepper, M., Greene, D., & Nisbett, R. (1973). Undermining children's intrinsic interest with extrinsic rewards: A test of the "overjustification" hypothesis. *Journal of Personality and Social Psychology, 28,* 129–137.

Letts, C., & Leinonen, E. (2001). Comprehension of inferential meaning in language impaired and language normal children. *International Journal of Language and Communication Disorders, 36,* 307–328.

Lin, L. C., & Johnson, C. (2005, June). *"Light and lamp are synonyms": Distributed characteristics of Taiwanese Mandarin-English bilingual preschoolers' semantic knowledge.* Paper presented at the Symposium on Research in Child Language Disorders, Madison, WI.

Lovaas, O. I., Berberich, J., Perloff, B., & Schaeffer, B. (1966). Acquisition of imitative speech by schizophrenic children. *Science, 151*(3711), 705–707.

Mackworth, N., Grandstaff, N., & Pribram, K. (1973). Orientation to pictorial novelty by speech-disordered children. *Neuropsychologia, 11,* 443–450.

MacWhinney, B. (1982). Basic syntactic processes. In S. Kuczaj (Ed.), *Language development: Syntax and semantics: Vol. 1.* (pp. 73–136). Hillsdale, NJ: Erlbaum.

Marcoux, C. (2004). *The cognitive advantage in bilingualism: Attention and working memory.* Unpublished master's thesis, University of British Columbia, Vancouver, British Columbia, Canada.

Margary, J. Retrieved June 26, 2005, from *The quotations page.* http://www.quotationspage.com/subjects/computers

Marler, J., Champlin, C., & Gillam, R. (2001). Backward and simultaneous masking measured in children with language-learning impairments who received intervention with Fast ForWord or Laureate Learning Systems software. *American Journal of Speech-Language Pathology, 10,* 258–268.

Mawhood, L., Howlin, P., & Rutter, M. (2000). Autism and developmental receptive language disorder—A comparative follow-up in early adult life, I: Cognitive and language outcomes. *Journal of Child Psychology and Psychiatry and Allied Disciplines, 41,* 547–559.

Mayer, R., & Anderson, R. (1991). Animations need narrations: An experimental test of a dual-coding hypothesis. *Journal of Educational Psychology, 83*(4), 484–490.

McCauley, R., & Swisher, L. (1984). Use and misuse of norm-referenced tests in clinical assessment: A hypothetical case. *Journal of Speech and Hearing Disorders, 49,* 338–348.

McGregor, K., Newman, R., Reilly, R., & Capone, N. (2002). Semantic representation and naming in children with specific language impairment. *Journal of Speech, Language, and Hearing Research, 45,* 998–1014.

Merzenich, M., Jenkins, W., Johnston, P., Schreiner, C., Miller, S., & Tallal, P. (1996). Temporal processing deficits of language-learning impaired children ameliorated by training. *Science, 271,* 77–81.

Miller, G. (1956). The magic number seven, plus or minus two: Some limits on our capacity for processing information. *Psychological Review, 63,* 81–97.

Miller, J. (1981). *Assessing language production in children.* Baltimore: University Park Press.

Miller, J. (1987). A grammatical characterization of language disorder. In *Proceedings of the first international symposium on specific speech and language disorders in children* (pp. 100–113). Brentford, UK: AFASIC.

Miller, J. (2004, October). *New approaches to language sample analysis.* Paper presented at the annual meeting of the British Columbia Association of Speech-Language Pathologists and Audiologists, Kelowna, BC.

Miller, J., & Iglesias, A. (2003–2005). Systematic analysis of language transcripts (SALT; Version 9) [Computer software]. Madison, WI: Language Analysis Laboratory, University of Wisconsin.

Miranda, A., McCabe, A., & Bliss, L. (1998). Jumping around and leaving things out: A profile of the narrative abilities of children with specific language impairment. *Applied Psycholinguistics, 19,* 647–667.

Moser, R. (2003). Beyond storage: *Working memory and specific language impairment.* Unpublished master's thesis, University of British Columbia, Vancouver, British Columbia, Canada.

Moser, R., & Johnston, J. (2004, June). *Beyond storage: Working memory and specific language impairment.* Paper presented at the Symposium on Research in Child Language Disorders, Madison, WI.

Munsch, R. (2000). *Mmm, Cookies!* New York: Scholastic.

Naigles, L., & Hoff-Ginsberg, E. (1995). Input to verb learning: Evidence for the plausibility of syntactic bootstrapping. *Developmental Psychology, 31,* 827–837.

Namazi, M. (1999). *Performance interactions and developmental asynchrony in the language of children with and without SLI.* Unpublished master's thesis, University of British Columbia, Vancouver, British Columbia, Canada.

Namazi, M., & Johnston, J. (1997, June). *Language performance and development in SLI.* Paper presented at the Symposium for Research in Child Language Disorders, Madison, WI.

Naremore, R. (1997). Making it hang together: Children's use of mental frameworks to structure narratives. *Topics in Language Disorders, 18,* 16–31.

National Institutes of Health. (2004). Central auditory processing disorder (Publication No. 01-4949). Retrieved June, 2005, from U.S. National Institute for Deafness and other Communication Disorders website, under Health Information: http://www.nidcd.nih.gov

Nelson, K. (1973). Structure and strategy in learning to talk. *Monographs of the Society for Research in Child Development, 38*(1–2, Serial No. 149).

Nelson, K. E. (1976). Facilitating children's syntax acquisition. *Developmental Psychology, 13,* 101–107.

Nelson, K. E., Camarata, S., Welsh, J., Butkovsky, L., & Camarata, M. (1996). Effects of imitative and conversational recasting treatment on the acquisition of grammar in children with specific language impairment and younger language-normal children. *Journal of Speech and Hearing Research, 39,* 850–859.

Newport, E., Gleitman, H., & Gleitman, L. (1977). Mother, I'd rather do it myself: Some effects and noneffects of maternal speech style. In C. Snow & C. Ferguson (Eds.), *Talking to children: Language input and acquisition* (pp. 109–149). Cambridge, MA: Cambridge University Press.

Norbury, C. (2005). Barking up the wrong tree: Lexical ambiguity resolution in children with language impairments and autistic spectrum disorders. *Journal of Experimental Child Psychology, 90,* 142–171.

Norbury, C., & Bishop, D. (2002). Inferential processing and story recall in children with communication problems. *International Journal of Language and Communication Disorders, 37,* 227–252.

Norman, D. (1976). *Memory and attention*. New York: Wiley.

Nye, C., Foster, S., & Seaman, D. (1987). Effectiveness of language intervention with the language/learning disabled. *Journal of Speech and Hearing Disorders, 52*, 348–357.

O'Brien, M., & Nagle, K. (1987). Parents' speech to toddlers: The effect of play context. *Journal of Child Language, 14*, 268–280.

O'Hara, M., & Johnston, J. (1997). Syntactic bootstrapping in children with specific language impairment. *European Journal of Disorders of Communication, 32*, 147–164.

Oldershaw, L. (2002). *A national survey of parents of young children*. Toronto: Invest in Kids.

Owens, R. (2001). *Language development* (5th ed.). Boston: Allyn and Bacon.

Oxelgren, C. (1998). *The dissociation of form and content in narrative development*. Unpublished master's thesis, University of British Columbia, Vancouver, British Columbia, Canada.

Oxelgren, C., & Johnston, J. (1996, November). *Cognitive aspects of narrative in children with specific language impairment*. Paper presented at the annual meeting of the American Speech-Language-Hearing Association, Seattle, WA.

Parkin, A., & Turcotte, A. (2004). *Bilingualism: Part of our past or part of our future?* Retrieved June, 2005, from Centre for Research and Information on Canada website, CRIC Papers: http://www.cric.ca

Parsons, C. (1991). *A comparison of two models of parent training in language intervention*. Unpublished master's thesis, University of British Columbia, Vancouver, British Colombia, Canada.

Paul, R. (1981). Analyzing complex sentence development. In J. F. Miller (Ed.), *Assessing language production in children* (pp. 67–71). Baltimore: University Park Press.

Paul, R. (1991). Late bloomers: Language development and delay in toddlers. *Topics in Language Disorders, 11*(4).

Paul, R., & Cohen, D. (1984). Outcomes of severe disorders of language acquisition. *Journal of Autism and Developmental Disorders, 14*, 405–421.

Peters, A. (1973). *The units of language acquisition*. Cambridge, UK: Cambridge University Press.

Piaget, J. (1962). *Play, dreams, and imitation* (C. Gattegno & F. Hodgson, Trans.). New York: Norton. (Original work published in 1951.)

Pinker, S. (1984). *Language learnability and language development*. Cambridge, MA: Harvard University Press.

Plomin, R., & Dale, P. S. (2000). Genetics and early language development: A UK study of twins. In D. Bishop & L. Leonard (Eds.), *Language impairments in children: Causes, characteristics, intervention, and outcome*. Hove, East Sussex, UK: Psychology Press.

Ramirez, J. D. (1998). *Performance of redesignated fluent-English-proficient students*. Retrieved June, 2005, from Annual Evaluation of SFSUD Language Academy by Center for Language Minority Education and Research, as presented on Language Policy website: http://ourworld.compuserve.com/homepages/JWCRAWFORD

Rapin, I. (Ed.). (1996). *Preschool children with inadequate communication*. London: MacKeith Press.

Rapin, I., & Allen, D. (1987). Developmental dysphasia and autism in preschool children. In *Proceedings of the first international symposium on specific speech and language disorders in children* (pp. 20–35). Brentford, UK: AFASIC.

Rapin, I., Allen, D., Aram, D., Dunn, M., Fein, D., Morris, R., et al. (1996). Classification issues. In I. Rapin (Ed.), *Preschool children with inadequate communication* (pp.190–213). London: MacKeith Press.

Rapin, I., & Dunn, M. (2003). Update on the language disorders of individuals on the autistic spectrum. *Brain and Development, 25*, 166–172.

Reggin, L. (2002). *Central executive functions in children with SLI*. Unpublished master's thesis, University of British Columbia, Vancouver, British Columbia, Canada.

Reggin, L., & Johnston, J. (2003, June). *Central executive functions in children with SLI*. Paper presented at the Symposium on Research in Child Language Disorders, Madison, Wisconsin.

Rescorla, L. (1989). The language development survey: A screening tool for delayed language in toddlers. *Journal of Speech and Hearing Disorders, 54*, 587–599.

Rispoli, M., & Hadley, P. (2001). The leading edge: The significance of sentence disruptions in the development of grammar. *Journal of Speech, Language, and Hearing Research, 44*, 1131–1143.

Roberts, J., Rice, M., & Tager-Flusberg, H. (2004). Tense marking in children with autism. *Applied Psycholinguistics, 25*, 429–448.

Robertson, S. (2004, November). *Using sign to facilitate expressive vocabulary in Late Talkers*. Paper presented at the annual conference of the American Speech-Language-Hearing Association, Philadelphia, PA.

Robertson, S., & Ellis-Weismer, S. (1997). The influence of peer models on the play scripts of children with specific language impairment. *Journal of Speech, Language, and Hearing Research, 40*, 49–61.

Rosenthal, W., Eisenson, J., & Luckau, J. (1972). A statistical test of the validity of diagnostic categories used in childhood language disorders: Implications for assessment procedures. *Papers and Reports in Child Language Development, 4*, 121–143.

Ross, D., & Ross, S. (1978). Facilitative effect of mnemonic strategies on multiple-associate learning in EMR children. *American Journal of Mental Deficiency, 82*, 460–466.

Ruder, K., & Smith, M. (1974). Issues in language training. In R. Schiefelbusch & L. Lloyd (Eds.), *Language perspectives: Acquisition, retardation, and intervention* (pp. 565–606). Baltimore: University Park Press.

Ruff, H., & Capozzoli, M. (2003). Development of attention and distractibility in the first four years of life. *Developmental Psychology, 39,* 877–890.

Sandhofer, C., Smith, L., & Luo, J. (2000). Counting nouns and verbs in the input: Differential frequencies, different kinds of learning? *Journal of Child Language, 27,* 561–585.

Scarborough, H. (1990). Index of productive syntax. *Applied Psycholinguistics, 11,* 1–22.

Scarborough, H., & Dobrich, W. (1990). Development of children with early language delay. *Journal of Speech and Hearing Research, 33,* 70–83.

Schery, T. (1985). Correlates of language development in language disordered children. *Journal of Speech and Hearing Disorders, 50,* 73–83.

Schminky, A., & Baran, J. (2000, Spring). CAPD: An overview of assessment and management practices. *SeeHear,* 41–52.

Scientific Learning Corporation. (1997–2005). Fast ForWord [Computer software]. Oakland, CA.

Serratrice, L. (2005). An interview with Annette Karmiloff-Smith. *Child Language Bulletin, 25,* 6–9.

Sevostianov, A., Fromm, S., Nechaev, V., Horwiz, B., & Braun, A. (2002). Effect of attention on central auditory processing: An fMRI study. *International Journal of Neuroscience, 112,* 586–606.

Shirai, Y., & Anderson, R. (1995). The acquisition of tense aspect morphology. *Language, 71,* 743–762.

Shonkoff, J., & Phillips, D. (Eds.). (2000). *From neurons to neighborhoods: The science of early childhood development.* Washington, DC: National Academy Press.

Siller, M., & Sigman, M. (2002). The behaviors of parents of children with autism predict the subsequent development of their children's communication. *Journal of Autism and Developmental Disorders, 32,* 77–89.

Simmons, N., & Johnston, J. (2003, February). *East Indian and Euro-Canadian mothers' beliefs and practices concerning talk to children.* Paper presented at the Early Years Conference, Vancouver, Canada.

Simons, H. (1996) The paradox of case study. *Cambridge Journal of Education, 26,* 225–240.

Slobin, D. (1973). Cognitive prerequisites for the development of grammar. In C. Ferguson & D. Slobin (Eds.), *Studies of child language development* (pp. 175–208). New York: Holt, Reinhart and Winston.

Smith, L. (2001). How domain-general processes may create domain-specific biases. In M. Bowerman & S. Levinson (Eds.), *Language acquisition and conceptual development* (pp. 101–131). Cambridge, UK: Cambridge University Press.

StatsCanada. (2002). *Profile of language in Canada*. Retrieved June, 2005, from Statistics Canada Website, 2001 Census Analysis Series at http://www12.statcan.ca

Stennes, L., Burch, M., Sen, M., & Bauer, P. (2005). A longitudinal study of gendered vocabulary and communicative action in young children. *Developmental Psychology, 41*, 75–88.

Stothard, S., Snowling, M., Bishop, D., Chipchase, B., & Kaplan, C. (1998). Language impaired preschoolers: A followup into adolescence. *Journal of Speech, Language, and Hearing Research, 41*, 407–418.

Stromswold, K. (2001). The heritability of language: A review and meta-analysis of twin, adoption, and linkage studies. *Language, 77*, 647–723.

Sturn, A., & Johnston, J. (1999). Thinking out loud: The use of problem-solving speech by children with language impairment. *International Journal of Language and Communication Disorders, 43*, 1–16.

Swanson, L., Trainin, F., & Necoechea, D. (2003). Rapid naming, phonological awareness, and reading: A meta-analysis of the correlation evidence. *Review of Educational Research, 73*, 407–440.

Tallal, P., Hirsch, L., Realpe-Bonilla, T., Miller, S., & Brzustowicz, L. (2001). Familial aggregation in specific language impairment. *Journal of Speech, Language, and Hearing Research, 44*(5), 1172–1182.

Tallal, P., Miller, S. L., Bedi, G., Wang, X., & Nagarajan, S. S. (1996). Language comprehension in language-learning impaired children improved with acoustically modified speech. *Science, 271*(5245), 81–84.

Tannen, D. (1990). *You just don't understand: Women and men in conversation*. New York: Ballantine.

Tannock, R., & Girolametto, L. (1992). Reassessing parent-focused language intervention programs. In S. Warren & J. Reichle (Eds.), *Causes and effects in communication and language intervention* (pp. 49–79). Baltimore, MD: Brookes.

Teitel, J. (2003). Is Jean Chrétien the greatest politician ever? *Saturday Night, 118*.

Thordardottir, E. (2002, November). *Parents' views on language impairment and bilingualism*. Paper presented at the annual meeting of the American Speech-Language-Hearing Association, Chicago, IL.

Thordardottir, E., Ellis Weismer, S., & Smith, M. (1997). Vocabulary learning in bilingual and monolingual clinical intervention. *Child Language Teaching and Therapy, 13*, 215–227.

Thordardottir, E., Rothenberg, A., & Rivard, M. E. (2003, June). *Effect of bilingual exposure on measures of receptive and expressive vocabulary and syntax*. Paper presented at the Symposium on Research in Child Language Disorders, Madison, WI.

Tomasello, M. (Ed.). (2003). *The new psychology of language: Cognitive and functional approaches to language structure, Vol 2*. Mahwah, NJ: Earlbaum.

Tomblin, J. B., Freese, P., & Records, N. (1992). Diagnosing specific language impairment in adults for the purposes of pedigree analysis. *Journal of Speech and Hearing Research, 35*, 832–843.

Trabasso, T., & Van den Broek, P. (1985). Causal thinking and the representation of narrative events. *Journal of Memory and Language, 24*, 612–630.

Trehub, S., & Henderson, J. (1996). Temporal resolution and subsequent language development. *Journal of Speech, Language, and Hearing Research, 39*, 1315–1320.

Tyler, A., Lewis, K., Haskill, A., & Tolbert, L. (2002). Efficacy and cross domain effects of a morphosyntax and phonological intervention. *Language, Speech, and Hearing Services in Schools, 33*, 52–66.

Tyler, A., Lewis, K., Haskill, A., & Tolbert, L. (2003). Outcomes of different speech and language goal attack strategies. *Journal of Speech, Language, and Hearing Research, 46*, 1077–1094.

Tyler, A., & Sandoval, K. (1994). Preschoolers with phonological and language disorders: Treating different linguistic domains. *Language, Speech, and Hearing Services in Schools, 25*, 215–234.

Uwer, R., Albrecht, R., & Von Suchodoletz, W. (2002). Automatic processing of tones and speech stimuli in children with specific language impairment. *Developmental Medicine and Child Neurology, 44*, 527–532.

van Kleeck, A. (1994). Potential cultural bias in training parents as conversational partners with their children who have delays in language development. *American Journal of Speech-Language Pathology, 3*(1), 67–78.

Vendler, Z. (1957). Verbs and times. *The Philosophical Review, 66*, 143–160.

Vig, S., & Jedrysek, E. (1999). Autistic features in young children with significant cognitive impairment: Autism or mental retardation? *Journal of Autism & Developmental Disorders, 29*, 235–248.

Vygotsky, L. (1962). *Thought and language*. Cambridge, MA: MIT Press.

Vygotsky, L. (1978). *Mind in society: The development of higher psychological processes*. Cambridge, MA: MIT Press.

Weber-Olson, M., & Ruder, K. (1984). Applications of developmental and remedial logic to language intervention. In K. Ruder & M. Smith (Eds.), *Developmental language intervention: Psycholinguistic applications* (pp. 231–270). Baltimore: University Park Press.

Weiss, A., Tomblin, J. B., & Robin, D. (1994). Language disorders. In J. B. Tomblin, H. Morris & D. Spriestersbach (Eds.), *Diagnosis in speech-language pathology* (pp. 99–134) San Diego: Singular.

Weissman, B. (2001). Letter to word court. *Atlantic Monthly, 288*(2), 144.

Wells, G. (1974). Learning to code experience through language. *Journal of Child Language, 1,* 243–269.

Wells, G. (1985). *Language development in the preschool years.* Cambridge: Cambridge University Press.

Wetherby, A., & Prizant, B. (2005). Enhancing language and communication development in autism spectrum disorders: Assessment and intervention guidelines. In D. Zager (Ed.), *Autism spectrum disorders: Identification, education, and treatment* (3rd ed., pp. 327–365). Mahwah, NJ: Erlbaum.

Whalen, C., & Schreibman, L. (2003). Joint attention training for children with autism using behavior modification procedures. *Journal of Child Psychology and Psychiatry, 44*(3), 456–468.

White, R. W. (1959). Motivation reconsidered: The concept of competence. *Psychological Review, 66,* 297–333.

Windfuhr, K., Faragher, B., & Conti-Ramsden, G. (2002). Lexical learning skills in young children with specific language impairment. *International Journal of Language and Communication Disorders, 37,* 415–432.

Wing, L. (1993). The definition and prevalence of autism: A review. *European Child and Adolescent Psychiatry, 2,* 61–74.

Yoder, P., Spruytenburg, H., Edwards, A., & Davies, B. (1995). Effect of verbal routine contexts and expansions on gains in the mean length of utterance in children with developmental delays. *Language, Speech, and Hearing Services in Schools, 26,* 21–32.

Young, A., Beitchman, J., Johnson, C., Douglas, L., Atkinson, L., Escobar, M., et al. (2002). Young adult academic outcomes in a longitudinal sample of early identified language impaired and control children. *Journal of Child Psychology and Psychiatry and Allied Disciplines, 43,* 635–646.

Yuill, N., & Oakhill, J. (1988). Effects of interference awareness training on poor reading comprehension. *Applied Cognitive Psychology, 2,* 33–45.

Author Index

Page numbers with a "t" or "f" denote tables and figures respectively.

Subject Index

Page numbers with a "t" or "f" denote tables and figures respectively.

A

ABA (Applied Behavioral Analysis), 170–73

alpha level judgments, 25–26

Ammon, Mary Sue, 117

analytic learners, 254–55

Applied Behavioral Analysis. *See* ABA

ASHA (American Speech-Language-Hearing Association), 14, 83, 85, 86–87

assessment
> differential diagnosis, 99–105, 106–13
> dynamic assessment, 126–31, 300
> local norms, 271–73
> measuring progress, 134–37
> narrative, 138–44, 149–51
> quantifiable vs. nonquantifiable aspects, 24–30
> standardized tests, 27–28, 97, 132–37, 291–94
> *See also* language sample analysis

asymptotic learning, 69–70, 141–42, 300

attention
> bilingualism and, 277–78
> CAPD and, 86
> development in, 173–75
> joint attention, 170–76, 213, 214
> selective attention, 93–94
> visual vs. auditory, 55, 64–65, 213, 214

auditory perception
> Fast ForWord, 27, 91–95, 256, 299
> language acquisition and, 5
> listening skills, 93–94
> perceptibility, 5
> SLI and, 85
> *See also* CAPD

auditory processing disorders. *See* CAPD

autism
> assessment approach comparison, 132–35
> change in definition, 99, 102, 113
> evidence-based practice, 11
> joint attention, 170–76
> motivators, 168–69
> vs. SLI, 106–13
> with/without language delay, 107–8

B

Baddeley, Alan, 53

Bamford Lahey Foundation, 14

bilingualism, 268–74, 275–80

bootstrapping, 6, 236–41, 245–48

bottom-up processing, 63

brain imaging, 44, 107, 110